The Horse Owner's Veterinary Handbook

Tony Pavord and Rod Fisher

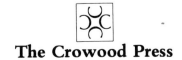

The Crowood Press

First published in 1987 by
The Crowood Press Ltd
Ramsbury, Marlborough,
Wiltshire SN8 2HR

This impression 1991

British Library Cataloguing in Publication Data

Pavord, Tony
  The horse owners veterinary handbook. — Rev. ed.
  1. Horses. Veterinary medicine
  I. Title   II. Fisher, Rod *1951*-.   III. Pavord, Tony.
  Equine veterinary manual
  636.1089

ISBN 1-85223-682-5

Acknowledgements

We wish to thank all who put up with us during the gestation
period of this book, especially our partner Collin Willson, and
our colleagues at Abbey Veterinary Centre. Our thanks also go
to those clients who, with great patience, allowed their horses to
pose for us. Our particular thanks go to Pam James, Marcy
Drummond and Susan Field who typed the manuscript, Dr Andy
Clarke for supplying Fig 24, and Andy Matthews for most of
the ophthalmic photographs.

Line illustrations by Elaine Roberts

Typeset by Alacrity Phototypesetters
Printed and bound in Great Britain by
BPCC Hazell Books, Aylesbury

Contents

Introduction

EVOLUTION OF THE HORSE

Some twenty million years ago a new plant family, Graminae, evolved. Very quickly, in evolutionary terms, the Graminae, which include the grasses, took advantage of the drier conditions existing in the northern hemisphere and colonised large areas. New grasslands were created, providing a plentiful food supply for any animal that could take advantage of it. The ancestor of the modern horse and his wild relatives, the zebra and ass, was such an animal. Over many millions of years *eohippus* changed from a small, cat-sized animal which lived in the dense forests of that time, to pony-sized *mesohippus*, superbly adapted to life on vast open plains.

These adaptations occurred in response to pressures exerted on the evolving horse by his new existence. Thus the teeth evolved into specialised cutters and grinders which enabled him to utilise the new tough grasses. Ears and eyes altered their shape and position to increase the acuteness of hearing and to widen the angle of vision during feeding. This development was necessary for survival, as the ability to scan a wide area, checking on the position of the herd and the presence of predators, was more important to the horse than the ability to examine the type of food just beyond his nose.

At the same time his limbs became adapted for sustained flight – the original legs, short and well-muscled, with five toes, became long, thin and single toed, with the propulsive power of the muscles concentrated at the top. These lighter, longer legs took less energy to move over the ground and flight could now be maintained over a greater distance. This process of change over many millions of years resulted in a species that was superbly adapted to a nomadic existence, constantly searching for new pastures and always alert to any danger.

MAN'S INTERVENTION

Three thousand years ago, a mere flicker in the period of time over which the horse has evolved, another successful species intervened. Man realised that this strong and speedy animal could be tamed and used to transport him and his goods from place to place. Over the last three thousand years, man has produced changes in the horse, by selective breeding, that are beyond measure.

Man's interference in the life of the horse is the cause of a variety of disorders and diseases. For example, we have the huge discrepancy in size that exists between the Welsh Mountain pony and the Shire horse, and we often ignore the congenital faults which our slavish regard for shape and type can produce.

We encourage the attitude that fatness and size are essential for successful showing, totally ignoring the fact that the excessive growth rate stimulated by overfeeding is positively harmful to the horse's health.

Immature youngsters are encouraged to become race-hardened athletes before their bones, joints and tendons are developed enough to cope with the stresses that are applied to them.

We expect our horses to cope with unnatural work-loads. The racehorse stands bored in his box for twenty-two hours, then works for two. The child's pony is confined to a box or small paddock all week and must then entertain a child, usually at maximum exertion, at weekends or during school holidays.

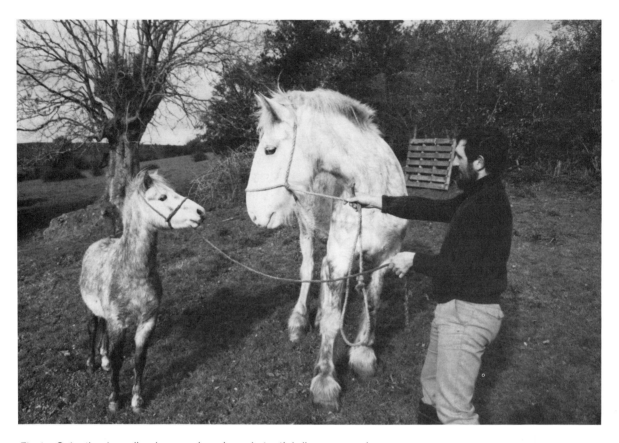

Fig 1   Selective breeding has produced a substantial discrepancy in size between the Welsh Mountain pony and the Shire horse.

Finally, we subject this gregarious species to a wide variety of environments. Grazing is often limited, so many parasite larvae are ingested. For our own convenience we expect the horse to remain housed for long periods, possibly in a dusty and badly ventilated box, and are then surprised when he develops a respiratory allergy or becomes a weaver. Conversely, large numbers of young horses, all strangers to one another, are herded together from different backgrounds, allowing an easy spread of infectious disease.

This catalogue of incidents demonstrates why man's treatment of the horse can cause such a variety of diseases. Hopefully our attempts in the following chapters to describe these diseases and the effects that they have on the horse will help to explain the pressures man puts on the horse and how we can minimise their adverse effects.

The emphasis throughout this book is on the way the horse's bodily systems work and how they react when something goes wrong. Little is said about treatment, as it is not the function of this book to be a 'do it yourself' vetting manual. Your horse should be too important to you to subject it to amateur doctoring, however well intentioned. What we do hope is that your increased knowledge of the workings of the horse and his response to injury and illness will enable you to care for him correctly and to judge when he does need the help and treatment of a veterinary surgeon.

1 The Healthy Horse

Before we worry about the many diseases and conditions which affect the sick horse, it is essential to recognise the normal, fit and healthy horse. For anyone who has owned a horse for some time, this is an intuitive reaction. We get used to his familiar nicker as we approach and the exuberant buck and canter as we let him out to pasture. When the nicker is absent and the buck and canter are replaced by a listless walk, our suspicions are aroused and the conscientious owner takes a more detailed look. Has all his hard food been eaten up? What are his droppings like? These questions and many more can provide the clues that, pieced together, tell us what is wrong.

GENERAL APPEARANCE

The healthy horse should be bright and alert at all times. His ears should be constantly moving to catch any interesting sound that might be coming his way and his eyes should be clear, with a moist salmon-pink conjunctiva (mucous membrane). In fact, all visible mucous membranes should be moist and a healthy pink colour. His coat should be glossy and the skin elastic. The muscles should be hard and clearly defined, not covered with a layer of fat, and the tendons should be cold with no bumps or swellings visible.

Watch how your horse gets up and down and how he moves. These actions should be free and supple, with his weight evenly distributed on all four legs. If one leg is rested more than the others, or if his weight is shifting from one foot to another, be warned. These may be signs that a lesion, a change which is due to injury or disease, is developing in the offending leg, or that some discomfort is being suffered, perhaps the first signs of abdominal pain or laminitis.

Remember that a horse is quite happy to lie asleep fully stretched, the picture of relaxation, but he can also rest standing up. We have all seen the position – head down, nodding, front legs slightly apart, one hind leg relaxed and the other locked at the patella, or kneecap, supporting the body weight. This position can be maintained for a long time with the weight supported by each hind leg alternately, and is most commonly seen during the lazy, hot, period around midday. However, this relaxed attitude should change to alert attention if a stranger approaches.

FEEDING

The horse's attitude to his feed can tell us a great deal about his state of health or ill health. Left to his own devices the horse prefers to feed little and often. His small stomach is emptied quickly and constant grazing is needed to keep it full. He has periods of grazing activity, generally during the morning and again in the evening, and periods of rest during the heat of the day. This method of feeding, coupled with the horse's inquisitive .nature, means that titbits are always accepted and a failure to do so can be a sign that all is not well.

The way a horse eats and drinks can also tell us much about his state of health. A horse uses his sensitive lips to convey food into his mouth. It is firstly nipped off by the incisor teeth, then chewed and broken up by the broad back teeth and guided into the oesophagus (the gullet) by the tongue and soft palate. Water is sucked into the mouth and down the oesophagus in the same smooth deliberate way.

PARAMETER		AVERAGE VALUE	RANGE
Respiration rate (per minute)		10	6–18
Heart rate (per minute)		42	28–64
Temperature	Degrees F	100.5	±1
	Degrees C	37.9	±0.3
Total blood volume (litres)		35	27–46
Total number of red blood cells (per litre)	Thoroughbreds in training	9 ($\times 10^{12}$)	7–11 ($\times 10^{12}$)
	other horses	7.5 ($\times 10^{12}$)	6–10.5 ($\times 10^{12}$)
Haemoglobin level (grammes per decilitre)	thoroughbreds in training	14	11–17.5
	other horses	11	9–15.5
Total white blood cells (per litre)		9 ($\times 10^{9}$)	5.5–12 ($\times 10^{9}$)
Neutrophils (per litre)		5.5 ($\times 10^{9}$)	2.5–7.5 ($\times 10^{9}$)
Lymphocytes (per litre)		3.5 ($\times 10^{9}$)	1.5–5.5 ($\times 10^{9}$)
Total faeces (kilogrammes per day)		17.5	10–30
Total urine (litres per day)		5	3–9

Fig 2 Some normal values in the average horse.

Any interruption in this efficient process may indicate a problem. Perhaps the teeth need attention, or maybe there is damage to the back of the throat, interfering with the passage of food on its way to the stomach. Some diseases, such as tetanus and grass sickness, have a specific effect upon mastication and swallowing, and early recognition of these signs means an early diagnosis.

As the food is digested, the large and small intestines move about in the abdominal cavity. Gases gurgle from one place to another and water and intestinal contents pass through the gut. The increase in the rate and intensity of gut sounds during an attack of spasmodic or flatulent colic is marked; the reverse is true during cases of impaction, when gut sounds become minimal. It is a good idea to familiarise yourself with the surprisingly loud, normal sounds which can be clearly heard with your ear held close to the horse's abdomen.

The quantity and consistency of the faeces and the colour and thickness of the urine also provide clues to the health status of your horse. Contrary to popular belief, the horse's urine can vary from a watery, pale yellow fluid to a thick, dark amber substance. It can be clear or cloudy and, depending on how much water the horse needs, the quantity passed each day can vary from two litres up to about four and a half litres (or from a few pints to more than a gallon). Similarly, the faeces can vary in consistency, from bright green, semi-solid cow pats, when the diet consists of fresh spring grass, to small, hard bullets when the diet is mostly grain and cake with a minimum of hay. However, diarrhoea, or soft, bad smelling faeces, is not normal and the reason for the change should be investigated at once. The quantity of faeces passed each day depends upon the size of the horse and the type of food being eaten. As a rough guide, a horse passes 2 per cent of its bodyweight as faeces each day about 12kg (26lb) a day for the average hunter.

The normal functions of the horse, those of eating, sleeping, moving and defecating, should become completely familiar to you so that any change in the horse's behaviour is recognised and acted upon. Physical signs should also be checked to see that they are normal, as they may reveal the reason for a change in behaviour.

TEMPERATURE

The body temperature is an important parameter and should be the first checked. In the horse, the normal temperature is 38C (100-100.5F). This should be measured with the horse at rest, as the temperature can rise quite normally after exercise.

Taking the temperature is not the easy matter that it seems when you watch your vet do it. First, check that you can see the magnified line of mercury running along inside the glass tube. It should be below the 35C (95F) mark. If it is not, shake it down, giving the thermometer quite a snap to ensure that the mercury column shortens into the bulb. Digital thermometers are available as an alternative, which, although accurate and easy to read, are rather expensive. Second, gently insert the thermometer into the rectum and leave it there for about a minute, before removing it and reading the temperature. It is just as well to hold on to the end of the thermometer; it is surprisingly difficult to remove a thermometer from the rectum after an anal contraction has sucked it in. Any rise in the temperature beyond 38C (100.5F) indicates that the horse is running a fever.

PULSE

The pulse, or the rate at which the heart is beating, is another parameter that is used to determine the well-being of the horse, although you, the owner, will more usually want to know your horse's heart rate if you

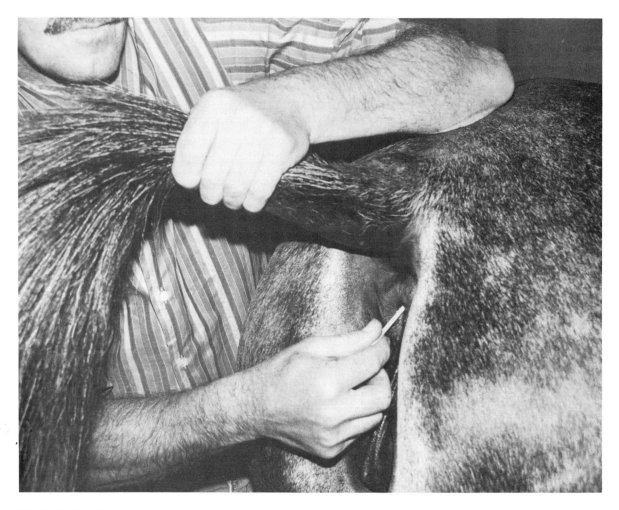

Fig 3   Taking the temperature.

take part in endurance riding. The heart rate can indicate how a horse is recovering from the work it has done and whether it is fit enough to continue. It is essential that you are able to monitor the heart rate, so that you get to know the recovery rate of your horse, both during training and competition.

The heart rate is best measured using a stethoscope, with the ear-pieces placed firmly in your ears and the head of the stethoscope placed on your horse's chest just behind the elbow. In this position, the typical heart sound 'luub–dup', repeated on average 40 times a minute, can be heard. In the normal horse the rate can vary from 32 to 52 beats a minute, and any strange or worrying stimulus can temporarily push the rate up another 10 to 20 beats. During strenuous exercise the rate can exceed 200 beats a minute.

The heart rate can also be measured by counting the pulse, the best place being just inside the angle of the jaw. A small artery passes over the bone at this point and with a little practice it is possible to feel the pulse as the blood is forced through this artery, past your fingers.

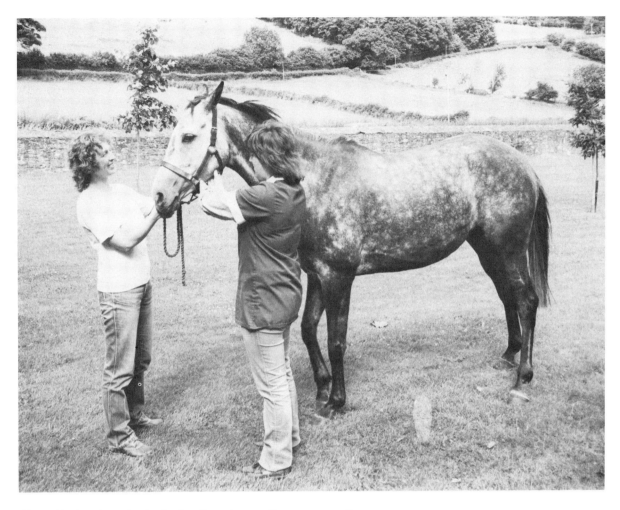

Fig 4   Taking the pulse by feeling the artery as it passes over the jaw-bone.

RESPIRATION

The rate at which a horse breathes, the respiration rate, can also indicate whether all is well. The horse normally takes between 8 and 16 breaths a minute, which can be observed by watching the flank move up and down or by feeling each breath as it is expelled from the nostrils. On a cold morning this is no trouble, as each expelled breath is visible as a cloud of vapour. Care should be taken if the rate of breathing is used as the sole indicator of ill health, as during hot weather the horse will pant in order to keep cool and will often sniff the air as he tests the interesting scents floating by.

The fascinating thing about the horse is that an infinite variety of moods and behaviour patterns go to make up the 'normal' animal. Before delving into the rest of this book to learn about abnormal conditions, you should make sure that the normal horse, how he feels, looks and sounds, is quite familiar to you.

2 You and Your Vet

A good relationship between vet and client should be based on trust, good humour, respect and a recognition of mutual dependence. Vets consider this relationship one of the most difficult but rewarding to achieve. The reasons are many, but the most important factor is the special bond between horse and owner. The horse, being half pet, half worker, invokes a more emotional response than a commercial farm animal. Any judgement involving the horse is therefore bound to be more difficult than the purely economic appraisal given to the farm animal.

From the veterinary surgeon's point of view, the immediate problem is to relate to his patient – only later does he begin to realise that there is a very anxious owner standing at the horse's head, wondering why the vet is taking such a long time. It is now that a sympathetic vet turns to his client and explains his diagnosis, the prognosis and any treatment needed.

From the client's point of view, the interference of an outsider in the bond between horse and owner is bound to cause apprehension. If basic communication with the vet has broken down, this becomes ten times worse.

As the case progresses, hopefully to a successful conclusion, the dialogue between vet and owner continues. Slowly a fragile relationship develops, the owner realising that the vet is doing his best, and the veterinary surgeon that the client is beginning to trust his judgement.

What, then, does each party expect of the other? Let us take the veterinary surgeon's point of view first.

1. Veterinary practice provides a 24 hour service, every day for the whole year. This does not mean that your favourite vet in the practice is on duty at all times (he has to relax some of the time), but it does mean that there is always a vet on the end of a phone. It helps to be sure that calls requested out of hours are necessary, and that non-urgent calls are phoned in as early in the morning as possible. If you have an urgent call, make sure that the staff at the surgery realise this. An urgent case will be dealt with by the nearest vet, but once the emergency is over, the case can be handed over to your own vet.

2. When the vet arrives, have ready a concise history of the problem, what the horse has had to eat and, most important, any drugs you may have given.

3. The vet would like his client to believe in his diagnosis and treatment. He expects any subsequent treatment to be carried out correctly, and to be notified if it is not working, or is impossible to administer. It is amazing how often a check-up examination reveals that the treatment prescribed has not been given because the horse would not eat it, or played up too much to be given an injection. No wonder some conditions take so long to clear up. It is more sensible to admit that you cannot give the injections prescribed; an alternative method can always be found.

Remember that it is impossible to treat some conditions. There are injuries that are too serious to remedy, some diseases which are incurable, and the cost of treating the horse that is not insured may be beyond the reach of you, the owner.

These possibilities should be discussed at the first examination but, because of their unwelcome nature, they are often neglected. It is an unpleasant fact of life that the more serious the condition, the less likely the recovery. As long as this is clearly understood from the beginning, the developing relationship between vet and client will not suffer.

4.   Delay in calling the vet is a false economy. If the case is seen as early as possible, not only is a diagnosis made more easily, but the treatment is simpler and more effective.

5.   Payment is a thorny subject – rarely mentioned by vet or client – and a facet of the relationship most likely to cause trouble. Why? Only too often a client is presented with a bill which to him seems excessive. Conversely, the veterinary surgeon considers it to be reasonable considering his expertise and technical back-up.

No accounting system is perfect, and genuine mistakes happen. The wrong job gets entered into the system, or the right job against the wrong client. The charge may not have been explained fully at the original examination, or late laboratory fees may have been charged after the original bill was sent. The errors which may occur are endless and rapidly become a recipe for disaster; the client withholds payment, and the vet chases it. It should be stressed that with good communication, a misunderstanding can be cleared up and mistakes rectified.

6.   Inevitably trust and respect sometimes break down. If they do, please tell your veterinary surgeon. He may sense when his client is unhappy with his conduct of a case and may suggest calling in a second opinion. This is much better for the patient, as both clinicians can then freely discuss the problem and prescribe the most effective treatment.

Looking at the relationship from the other side, what does the owner want from his vet? Confidence in his ability to examine, diagnose and treat the patient must lie high on the list.

1.   Check that the vet you are considering is, in fact, used to horses, rather than the cheapest in the area or the nearest, who may be an expert in the treatment of small animals but who may know little about horse problems. Word of mouth recommendation is the best way of choosing your vet.

2.   A professional appearance is important to some people. However, first impressions can be unreliable and the attitude and general approach to the patient is of more value.

3.   The vet should handle the horse with firmness and kindness, and show that he has an empathy with the equine species. Equally, the vet would like his patient to be reasonably well behaved. We expect a certain reluctance on the part of the patient when confronted with needles, stomach tubes and other unpleasant procedures, but the horse should not act up during a normal examination.

4.   At the end of the consultation, the client should expect to be told clearly and concisely the cause of the disease or injury, the prognosis and, as has already been pointed out, the need for and cost of treatment. A clear appreciation of the problem on the part of the client makes for a more enthusiastic and capable approach to the long period of care and nursing which some cases need.

If you feel that a full explanation has not been given or that you are confused, ask. Veterinary surgeons often assume that because they understand the condition, the owner does too, by some miraculous thought transference. The resultant discussion is of great value, adding to mutual understanding and developing the relationship.

In conclusion, we would reiterate that a good relationship is based on trust, good humour and a realisation of mutual dependence. Another quality – tolerance – might easily be added. If all these are present, then you, your horse and your vet can look forward to a rewarding relationship.

3 Veterinary Examinations

In the course of their working day, veterinary surgeons are asked to perform many different types of examination on apparently normal horses.

THE PURCHASE EXAMINATION

It must be a compliment to the veterinary profession that the word 'to vet' has been incorporated into the English language as a term meaning 'to examine critically'. For many years it has been the custom for a vet to check that a horse is sound before a potential buyer takes the plunge and parts with his or her money. But what does the term 'sound' mean? In these litigation-conscious days, it is almost impossible to define and, as a term, it is of little value.

If you understand a 'sound' horse to be one with no faults at all then such horses are a rarity indeed; the cost of searching for one would quickly become prohibitive and the frustration enormous. So how do you overcome this problem? One answer is to assume that no horse is perfect. The examination then becomes an assessment of the health status of the horse together with medical abnormalities. It is necessary for the significance of these abnormalities to be explained, by the examining vet, to the prospective buyer.

Whether an abnormality renders the horse unsuitable for purchase depends on the purpose for which the horse is intended. To take extreme examples, a horse who is permanently lame with a limb injury is unlikely to be of any use at all. In contrast, a horse who has been castrated, while clearly unsuitable for breeding purposes, could be quite functional as a race-horse, eventer or riding horse.

It follows, therefore, that a vet can not make an examination on behalf of the person selling the horse, which would then be reported to a prospective buyer. It would be human nature for the vet in this situation to minimise or even overlook abnormalities as being of no significance; he may even fail to explain fully their implications to the buyer.

The vet can easily be placed in an invidious position, if both vendor and potential purchaser are his clients, particularly where he knows that the horse has previously had problems. Provided that he is fair to the potential purchaser, it is permissible to complete the examination. However, if your vet declines to carry out an examination on your behalf simply because the vendor is also his client, do not automatically assume that there is something wrong with the horse.

The examination is an assessment of the horse only on the day on which he was examined and it is not a guarantee of his future health. The vet cannot be expected to gaze into a crystal ball. However, if a problem develops in the future due to an abnormality which was missed or not fully explained at the original examination, then the examining vet is at fault.

Normally the examination is made with the help of simple aids, a stethoscope to listen with and an ophthalmoscope to look with. Attempts to extend the scope of the examination have been made by using specialised techniques. On the whole, however, this introduces more problems than it solves.

The problems lie in the interpretation of the results of these techniques. The one technique commonly in use is X-ray. Radiography is used particularly to detect navicular disease, but also on areas besides the feet to detect hitherto unsuspected orthopaedic problems. By definition, however, a horse cannot be diagnosed as having navicular disease unless it is lame. The radiographic changes that accompany navicular disease may even be present in horses who do not have, and possibly never will have, navicular disease. Thus, although the horse is sound and in all probability will remain so, the radiographic evidence has an influence on whether to buy or not. This is not a satisfactory situation.

Another unfortunate and increasing problem that has to be faced, is the use of drugs, generally pain-killers, to mask a condition which might become evident during the purchase examination. The most common reason for this would be to hide lameness. Where it is suspected for some reason that drugs have been administered for this purpose, it is possible, but not a routine procedure, to take a blood sample, with the owner's agreement. This can be analysed for undisclosed substances but clearly would add considerably to the cost of the examination.

Vices are a problem area, since they are considered an unsoundness, but frequently cannot be detected at the time of the examination. Normal practice is to rely on a declaration made by the vendor, that the horse is free of all vices. This is held to be legally binding.

Often clients request that only a partial examination be made, presumably with the aim of cutting costs. How far does this partial examination go? To examine the heart and lungs at rest tells us very little about their ability to work under stress. Equally, it is unacceptable to state that a horse is sound in action when the only action seen is a trot in hand. Consequently, even to cover these areas, a prolonged examination must be made, and the cost of such an examination will still be relatively high. A partial examination will inevitably lead to argument as to what areas have been covered, especially if, in the future, a fault develops in one of those areas. As a result, such an examination must be considered in-

adequate.

Bearing these points in mind, it becomes clear that whether your horse is sound or not is by no means a clear-cut 'yes' or 'no' assessment. Every horse is worth something even if only its carcass value. What you must decide, when your vet makes his report, is whether you are prepared to buy the horse despite the faults which he has found, and if so, at what price? Your vet cannot help you to name a price. He is not a horse valuer and the amount that you are prepared to pay is governed entirely by how much you want the horse, which only you can know.

THE INSURANCE EXAMINATION

Our knowlege of disease and our ability to cure it is increasing constantly, as are the surgical techniques available to cope with bone fractures and accidents. Unfortunately this increasing expertise costs money for materials, professional skill and the expense of convalescence. In order to protect the horse and themselves, more and more owners are taking out an insurance policy to cover this risk.

One of the necessary examinations that the vet carries out is the one that he does on behalf of the insurance companies. Before accepting the risk of insuring the health and life of a horse, the insurance company wants to know whether the horse is what he is stated to be and that he is in good health and a suitable insurance risk. As the insurance companies are facing a rising level of claims, they are demanding, quite rightly, a more comprehensive insurance examination. No longer are they satisfied with a visual inspection; the examination now approaches the thoroughness of a purchase examination.

IDENTIFICATION EXAMINATIONS

Horses need to be identified. Some breed societies require that their breeding stock be blood typed and identified, and the racing industry, through Wetherbys, organises a most comprehensive identification system. Veterinary surgeons find that they have to examine many horses and positively identify them by recording on a chart the distribution of their hair patterns or whorls, any white areas and the position of any permanent scars. A detailed written description is made at the same time.

It is important to realise that this document is used to identify the horse for the rest of his life, so the identification examination must be very comprehensive. It is no use bringing the youngster in, unhandled and unwashed, with his coat a mass of knots and mud-caked hair. It is impossible to describe such an animal accurately. A plea from all vets involved in such examinations would be to have the foal or yearling presented in hand, clean and in good light.

LOCAL AUTHORITY EXAMINATIONS

In order to run a riding establishment, or, as the Riding Establishment Act, 1970, defines it, 'the carrying on of a business of the keeping of horses to let them out on hire for riding, or for use in providing instruction for payment, or both', a licence issued by the local authority is needed. Before this licence is issued, the premises and the horses have to be inspected by a veterinary surgeon appointed by the local authority, and judged to be of a suitable standard for the purpose.

THE EXAMINATION FOR THE JOINT MEASUREMENT SCHEME

The Joint Measurement Scheme was set up nationally to measure the height of horses and ponies in order that they could be identified and classified for competition.

The examination is carried out by a veterinary surgeon who is appointed to the panel on a yearly basis. Two types of certificate can be issued.

Annual Certificates

Annual Certificates can be issued to horses who are 4 and 5 years old and to any horse of 6 years and over being examined for the first time. The age is worked out from January. A horse is 1 year old on 1 January after the year of birth.

When the horse is measured for a second Annual Certificate, the measurement must be carried out by a different vet although he may be from the same practice.

Life Certificates

The Life Certificate is issued to horses 6 years and over, who already hold an Annual Certificate. The vet who carries out this examination must be from a different practice from that of the Official Measurer who performed the last Annual Certificate.

Anyone competing in international events under FEI rules (Federation Equestre Internationale) should check the FEI requirements if a height certificate is needed.

The Measurement Examination

The measurement should take place on a suitable smooth, hard, level area at least 3m by 1m in size. The area should be in a place where the horse can relax. These requirements are so difficult to fulfil that Official Measurers now insist that the horse be brought to and measured on their own measuring pad, which they know to be suitable. After 1 January 1987 only Joint Measurement Scheme registered pads may be used.

The horse should be without shoes and the feet should be trimmed and balanced, as if about to be shod. The hair over the withers should be removed.

The first part of the examination is taken up by completing the diagram and written description of the horse. If the animal has been measured before, the description is checked to ensure that positive identification can be made. The time taken to complete this procedure is used to let the horse get used to his surroundings and relax. It is not generally realised that the horse can lose as much as an inch in height as the muscles relax.

The position of the horse as it is measured is important. The rule book *Joint Measurement Scheme Rules,* obtainable from the Joint Measurement Scheme Limited, British Equestrian Centre, Kenilworth, Warwickshire CV 8 2LR., states that:

the horse should stand with its front legs perpendicular and parallel with the toes in line. Both hind limbs should be taking weight and as near to the perpendicular as possible, the toes should be no more than 6 inches out of line. The head should be in a natural position with the eyes not more or less than 3 inches above or below the level of the withers.

The measurement is taken at the highest point of the withers, which is immediately above the spinal process of the 5th thoracic vertebra. A measuring stick passed by a Weights and Measures Officer is used.

Re-measurement In the case of doubt or objection to the height of a horse, an arbitration procedure does exist. This allows for the remeasurement of the horse by two referees. Their decision concerning the height of the horse is final and binding.

4 Digestive System

Herbivores which rely on plant materials containing a high level of cellulose for a source of energy, require a large fermentation chamber in which the cellulose can be digested. In contrast to the ruminant cow or sheep, whose fermentation chambers are part of the stomach at the start of the alimentary canal, the horse's fermentation chamber is the caecum and large colon at the rear end of the gut.

MASTICATION

Food is collected in the mouth using very prehensile lips and the incisor teeth. It is ground between the cheek teeth and thoroughly mixed with saliva using tongue and jaw movements. Saliva is produced by the parotid and submaxillary salivary glands. Its production is stimulated by the movement of the jaw and, unlike in the dog, it cannot be produced as a conditioned response to the smell of food. Up to 50ml or about 0.09pt can be produced each minute. It is rich in bicarbonate but low in digestive power.

STOMACH

After thorough mixing the food is passed down the oesophagus or gullet to the stomach. The horse's stomach is comparatively very small, comprising only 9 per cent of the total volume of the alimentary canal. The total capacity is 10–15l (about 17–26pt) and reflects the horse's habit of continuous eating in that the stomach is rarely empty. In the foal the stomach functions in much the same way as in man or the dog, and food remains much longer in the stomach. In the adult horse bacterial fermentation is responsible for the production of lactic acid which is absorbed as a source of energy in the small intestine or converted into fatty acids in the large intestine. The horse's gut naturally contains a population of bacteria which process food during digestion. Fermentation is controlled by bicarbonate in the saliva. With saliva, secretions in the stomach amount to 10–30l (about 17–52pt) a day. The mechanical activity of the stomach is important; the slow and irregular movements after fasting become quicker and more regular after feeding.

Horses are normally unable to vomit, due to the very strong muscle at the inlet to the stomach. The stomach will rupture before the muscle relaxes. The normal pressure inside the stomach is $10g/cm^2$ but when gas builds up (tympany), pressure can reach $50g/cm^2$ and at $55-69g/cm^2$ the stomach ruptures.

SMALL INTESTINE

Food passes from the stomach into the small intestine where it is mixed with secretions from the adjacent pancreas. Pancreatic juice is profusely and continuously produced, with output being increased by nervous or hormonal stimulation. Compared with other species, the digestive enzyme content of the horse's pancreatic juice is low, but output is 5–12l (8.75–21pt) daily. Since the horse has no gall bladder, secretion of bile is continuous. These secretions contain much bicarbonate which renders the environment more alkaline.

The small intestine is 10–20m (about 32–64ft) long but has a vast surface area due to minute finger-like projections along the walls. Furthermore, the lining cells have borders

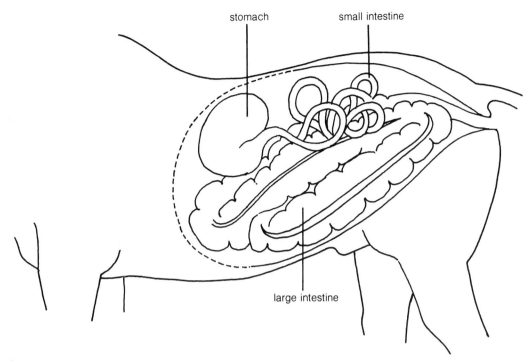

Fig 5 Structure of the digestive system (left side).

which resemble a brush, enormously increasing the surface area. These brush borders contain enzymes – chemicals which break down the food material. Enzymes known as disaccharidases digest sugars. At birth this is mainly lactose from milk. The ability to digest lactose reduces after four years of age and the ability to digest maltose and sucrose increases during sucking.

Alkaline phosphatase helps fat digestion and peptidases help digest proteins. Carbohydrate – the main source of energy – starts to be broken down here. Dietary grain has a high level of soluble carbohydrate. In all, 65 per cent of protein, 70 per cent of soluble carbohydrate, 20 per cent of fibre and fats, and certain minerals, particularly calcium and magnesium, are absorbed here. Glucose and galactose, a similar energy source, are absorbed from here and pass to the liver for use for energy, or to be converted into glycogen (a starch) or fats for storage.

CAECUM AND LARGE INTESTINE

From the small intestine the food has two alternatives. It can either pass directly into the large intestine or it can pass into the caecum. Unlike the non-functional, shrunken appendix which is the equivalent in man, the caecum in the horse is a huge and vital, blind ending fermentation chamber; elongated and pear shaped, it lies along the whole of the right side of the horse's abdomen.

Bacterial Action

The caecum and large intestine (colon) contain a variety of bacteria which are essential for the digestion of various food materials. Different bacteria work on different foods, particularly cellulose and lignin which form the walls of plant material. These bacteria enable herbivores to benefit nutritionally from these

15

materials where carnivores cannot. The bacteria are also responsible for producing vitamins, particularly of the B vitamin group. In addition, they are used to provide a variety of amino acids, the building blocks of proteins, as the horse can only form *some* amino acids himself.

The greatest variety of bacteria occurs in the caecum and the ventral colon. Their most important function is the conversion of plant material into volatile fatty acids, acetic, butyric and propionic acids which are readily absorbed energy sources.

Colon Position

The colon runs along the floor of the abdomen, from back to front on the right side, before doing a U-turn and returning along the left side. This sudden change in direction may be a site for material to become blocked, but a more common site is where the colon reaches the back of the abdomen again. Here, besides doing a turn through 180 degrees in the vertical plane, it suddenly narrows markedly so that an impaction at this point is fairly common under certain circumstances. The colon then returns along the top of the earlier portion of colon, completing a second U-turn at the front of the abdomen, widening again and finishing at the back of the abdomen on the right side. From here it again narrows rapidly and starts to form faecal boluses (balls of waste matter) which are passed to the rectum for storage. Food is moved along the colon by large contractions and smaller uncoordinated contractions and a pendular movement.

Water Reabsorption

Water passes across the gut wall in both directions along its length. 90 per cent of that which is passed into the gut is subsequently reabsorbed. The primary site for this reabsorption is in the colon. Slight changes in the ability to reabsorb water cause great changes in water loss. For example, damage to the cells of the gut wall which renders them 10 per cent less efficient means that instead of 90 per cent of fluid being reabsorbed, a little over 80 per cent is reabsorbed so that there is a 100 per cent increase in water loss. This explains why diarrhoea can cause such severe changes so quickly. Water intake is normally 35-45 litres a day but can be greatly increased during diarrhoea.

Normally faeces are passed eight to nine times daily, producing 10 to 20kg. This amount is increased when a high fibre diet is being fed or during diarrhoea. Food normally takes between 64-96 hours to pass right through the gut.

TEETH AND DENTAL CARE

Incisors

The horse has three pairs of incisor teeth in each jaw, which are used to collect food material into the mouth. The first pair of temporary teeth is usually present at birth or appears within the first week of life. By nine months all three pairs are present. These are small white teeth with a definite neck, in contrast to the larger, more square permanent teeth which replace them.

This replacement is fairly accurately timed. First the central pair is replaced, then the pair outside them, and finally the outer pair. Since these changes occur at two and a half, three and a half and four and a half years respectively, with the new teeth coming into wear six months later, the age of the horse up to five years of age can be very accurately determined from the incisor teeth. Beyond this age, more emphasis must be placed on the wearing surfaces of the teeth.

When the tooth erupts, the centre is hollow giving the tooth a shell-like appearance. This hole or infundibulum is tapered and so gradually reduces in size, first in the central teeth and then in the outer ones. As the infundibulum fades, it is replaced by a stain in the dentine that forms the central part of the tooth – the dental star. The dental star becomes progressively larger and darker in colour, again first in the central teeth. By about thirteen years, all the infundibula have disappeared. Overlapping with this process, at about ten years of age, a dark groove appears in the upper, outer incisors – Galvayne's groove. It grows steadily down the tooth until, by twenty years old, it has reached the biting (occlusal) surface, after which it grows out.

Meanwhile, the angle of the teeth in profile changes, from almost vertical in the young horse, reducing gradually to less than 120 degrees by twenty-five years of age. The shape of individual teeth changes in section from being flat and elongated, through square to triangular, and finally more elongated from front to back. The teeth also appear longer as the gums recede.

All these factors must be considered when trying to make an assessment of age. Beyond about eight years, the ability to assess age accurately reduces with time and also depends on the horse's diet. Obviously the coarser and more abrasive the diet, the faster the teeth will be worn.

Cheek Teeth

Continuous growth of the teeth, in contrast to those of man and the carnivores, is necessary. The nature of the horse's diet means that food must be well ground between the cheek (molar and premolar) teeth before being swallowed, to enable adequate digestion to take place. If food is not sufficiently ground, the full nutritional value is not obtained from it and the horse starts to lose weight.

The cheek teeth consist of three or four premolars on each side of each jaw, depending on whether wolf teeth are present, and a further three molars behind. The premolars are present first and are gradually replaced, the

process not being complete until three and a half years. Molars are not replaced, and they take from eight months to four years to appear.

DENTAL PROBLEMS

In the early stages, signs of teeth problems may be subtle – difficulty in mastication or chewing, characterised by an increase in the time taken to eat a set amount of food. 'Quidding' – the dropping of feed from the mouth during eating – is relatively rare. Pressure on the outside of the cheek, either from the hand or the bridle, may cause pain. Whole cereal may appear in the faeces since it has not been adequately ground, so is not properly digested. Where more serious problems are present there may be swelling of the face or a discharge from one nostril.

Sharpness

The reason why teeth become sharp relates to the relative positions of the teeth and the action of the jaws in mastication. The rows of teeth (dental arcades) are set 30 degrees further apart in the upper jaw (the maxilla) than in the lower jaw (the mandible). This means that the upper teeth overlap on the outside. When chewing, the horse moves the lower jaw in a vertical plane in relation to the maxilla, and in a circular motion from front to back (see fig 6). Consequently the areas in contact wear, while those that do not make contact develop sharp edges. Sharp edges occur on the inside (lingual) margin of the lower teeth and the outside (buccal) margin of the upper teeth. The overlying cheek may become ulcerated and painful. This pain is most obvious when bridle pressure is applied, particularly on turning. The horse tries to move forward with his head turned away from the affected side.

In addition, if the upper and lower jaws move apart before they reach the end of the opposing arcade, the end tooth may not be

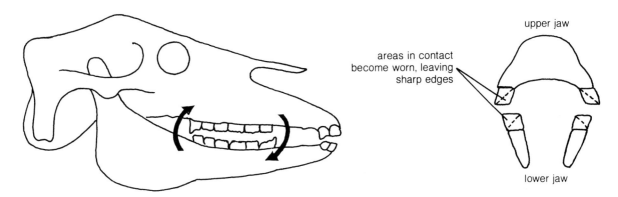

direction of movement of jaw during eating
hooks form where anterior/posterior occlusion is incomplete

Fig 6   Relative positions of the upper and lower jaw; where teeth are
in contact during mastication, sharp edges may be formed.

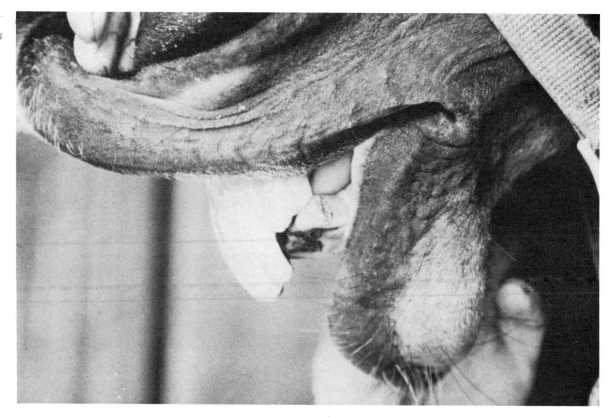

Fig 7   A severely undershot lower jaw, which does not affect eating
in this successful chaser.

adequately worn, resulting in the formation of a hook, or beak, on the upper, first cheek teeth and the lower, back cheek teeth, or vice versa. Hook formation is exacerbated in horses whose cheek teeth do not naturally lie opposite each other or whose upper jaws are longer or shorter than their lower jaws, producing parrot mouth or pig mouth respectively. Certain family lines are predisposed to hook formation.

Eruption

As the horse's teeth are worn away, they are replaced by further growth. Cheek teeth grow at the rate of 3mm per year. Eruption of the teeth occurs up to four and a half years of age, so that the period from two to five years of age is one of intense dental activity. The teeth should be checked twice annually during this period and once annually thereafter.

As the second or third cheek teeth erupt, they dislodge the overlying, temporary teeth which may then sit on the erupting tooth as a cap. This causes difficulty in eating and manual removal of the cap may be necessary.

Overcrowding is another potential problem during the main eruption period from two to four years. The result may be swellings in the region of the offending roots in the upper or lower jaws. Swellings over the roots of the mandibular teeth at the time of eruption (that is, along the bottom of the lower jaw) are normal. The swelling indicates that the tooth is growing at the root faster than it can erupt, so that it grows in both directions.

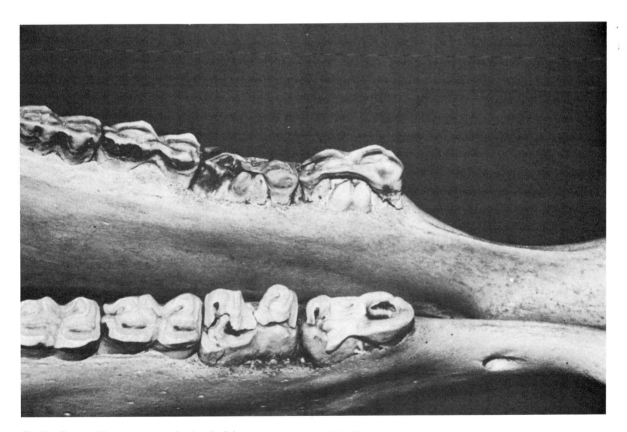

Fig 8 Caps of temporary molar teeth, lying over permanent teeth, can make eating difficult.

19

Infection

Infection of the tooth develops where opposing teeth do not meet closely, resulting in loosening, rotation and finally loss of the tooth. Tooth decay (caries) results from infection of the pulp cavity. Dentine has a higher protein content and so can be more easily broken down by certain bacteria. The cement lakes in the centre of the cheek teeth unite to form a line of mechanical weakness in which infection develops. In the upper jaw the cement may not be adequately developed in the first place. The third cheek teeth are the last to develop and are the most likely to be affected.

It is fortunate that infections of horses' teeth are uncommon, since treatment can be difficult. In the upper teeth, swelling of the face and a discharging sinus may result. The number of teeth involved in the infection is best assessed using X-ray and can be done more easily with the horse under general anaesthesia.

The extraction of affected teeth, to achieve drainage of the infected area, can be difficult. Only when there is gross disease, fracture of the tooth or a horse who is very old, can the affected tooth normally be removed via the mouth. More commonly it is necessary to approach the tooth through a hole in the bone and to punch the tooth from the jaw with the aid of a mallet and punch. The hole is made either with a circular saw (a trephine) or by cutting a flap in the bone, which is later replaced. Even then it is difficult, since the teeth roots are angled in the jaw and the roots must be approached at the correct angle. More than a quarter of treated horses subsequently require further surgery to remove small pieces of tooth which have been missed.

Canine Teeth

Canine teeth, or tushes, are not normally a problem. They are usually absent or rudimentary in female horses. They erupt at approximately four years of age and are not normally preceded by temporary canines. Because they are not in contact with opposing teeth, they often become covered with plaques of tartar which look unpleasant but seldom affect the horse. The canine teeth are situated in the diastema, the space, known as the bars, between the incisors and the cheek teeth, usually slightly nearer the incisors. They form the forward extremity of the bars of the mouth in which the bit is placed. They are often confused with wolf teeth.

Wolf Teeth

Wolf teeth are vestigial premolars which erupt at approximately six months and lie immediately in front of the cheek teeth. Frequently they are blamed as the cause of a horse fighting the bit and are therefore likely to cause most problems at about four or five years of age. Although they are often the scapegoat for faulty riding techniques or ill-fitting bridles, they do sometimes cause problems, particularly where the teeth are displaced forwards or to the side. The offending teeth can easily be removed.

Problem Prevention

Since most abnormalities of wear of the cheek teeth occur as a result of eating hard food, it is most logical to have the teeth checked during the spring period before grazing begins. This is best done with minimal restraint, but some fractious horses may require the use of a twitch or even sedation.

The teeth all need to be examined by testing the sharpness of the edges with the fingers. This can be done either by holding the tongue to one side with the other hand, or, more safely, by using a gag to hold the mouth open. A gag is essential if a careful examination of the last cheek teeth is to be made. Large hooks may need to be knocked off with a sharp, cold chisel and the remaining sharp edges and points may

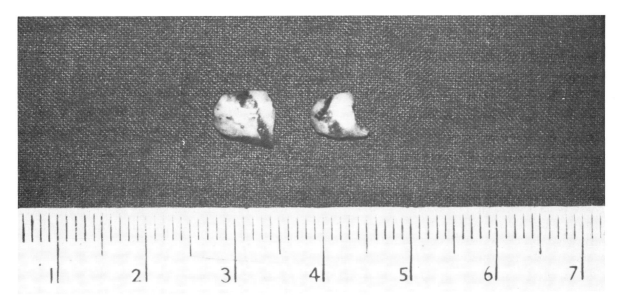

Fig 9   Wolf teeth, shown beside a scale calibrated in inches.

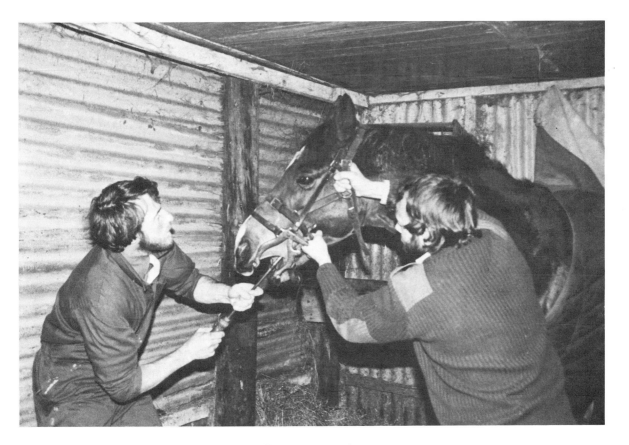

Fig 10   Teeth should be checked, and rasped if necessary, at least
once a year.

have to be removed by rasping or 'floating'. This reduces the incidence of irregular wear and minimises subsequent disease. Two floats are needed. A flat one reaches the surfaces of the cheek teeth of the lower jaw and the back cheek teeth of the upper jaw. To reach the front cheek teeth of the upper jaw, the blade must be angled to allow the rasp to pass the upper incisor teeth.

It is uncommon for the incisor teeth to require attention. Horses with quite severe parrot mouths can eat perfectly adequately.

Lampas Lampas is a normal state of the soft tissue overlying the hard palate behind the upper incisor teeth. The tissue overlaps the erupting incisor teeth between the ages of two and a half and four years. Many forms of treatment have been tried, but none is necessary apart from feeding soft food and avoiding sharp oat awns if the tissue is inflamed.

NUTRITIONAL DISORDERS

The normal preconception that the necessary diet of the horse consists of oats and hay or grass, while being very inflexible and by no means the only option, is based on generations of proven effectiveness and freedom from problems. This combination provides a diet which is relatively high in fibre and yet also supplies energy for performance. While many other feeds are perfectly suitable, it is difficult to know where their pitfalls lie, and how to avoid them. Several principles should be followed, but primarily you should avoid sudden changes in diet. All changes should be made slowly so that the bacteria in the intestines can adapt. This will prevent the dangers of diarrhoea and tympanitic (or flatulent) colic.

Fibre

The horse is naturally a browsing animal, eating little and often. Although adapted to a diet of vegetable fibre, he can survive without. The normal behaviour of frequent grazing provides an adequate food supply with no overloading of the system, but one problem is to maintain the appetite during extended periods of maximum work. In the working horse the diet must be artificially modified to allow the horse to work, by reducing his feeding time. To this end, herbage is replaced by cereals and their by-products, and by conserved dry grass (hay) or silage. The extent to which this can be done is limited.

Fibre is essential in the diet to provide bulk, since this promotes the waves of contraction on the gut (peristalsis) which push the food along, preventing blockage. However, too fibrous a diet, as occurs with straw or poor quality hay, may lead to impaction on the turning points of the intestine, described earlier.

The time available for eating and the quality of the fibre source, together with the requirement governed by the amount of work being done, dictates the quantity of cereal which will be needed to supplement the fibre. In considering the ratio of fibre to starch, it should be remembered that starch is digested primarily in the small intestine to produce mainly glucose, whereas fibre is digested in the hind gut to produce fatty acids. Organisms which ferment starch in the gut work faster than fibre fermenters so that they increase the rate of digestion and fermentation. Consequently, energy is more rapidly produced and may account for the excessive excitability commonly known as 'overheating', a misnomer which is best avoided since the body temperature is perfectly normal.

Cereals with high digestibility – maize, barley and wheat – allow a very rapid build-up of glycogen, and this factor may be significant in horses developing azoturia, where large amounts of glycogen are rapidly and inefficiently broken down. Oats have a lower digestibility since the fibrous coat is slowly digested, effectively diluting the feed value.

The lower energy level per unit weight means that more oats can be fed before problems arise.

Where the fibre content of the feed is high, more chewing is required before swallowing. As a result, more saliva is produced which in turn neutralises the acidity of the stomach to a greater extent. The saliva also aids passage of food. Wheat has a low fibre content; its gluten forms a pasty material in the gut and it is therefore an unsuitable food for horses.

Protein

All horses require protein to replace body tissues. Consequently, growing foals have a greater protein requirement than adult horses.

In adult horses, the quality of protein supplied is not important, but in the foal poor quality protein can have a severely adverse effect. Most proteins are limited in their content of lysine – a basic amino acid building block. Unlike the adult, the foal's hind gut is inadequately developed for the young animal to manufacture its own.

For the horse in work, the protein requirement is a constant, proportional to the energy requirement, and is surprisingly low. The use of non-protein nitrogen in the form of urea, as a cheap replacement for expensive protein, is not likely to be effective. It only works in rapidly growing youngstock in which the caecum has developed, and in lactating mares. However, the commonly held belief that excessive dietary protein poisons the horse is not likely to be true in practice. Finally, remember that leafy grass is high in protein, whereas older fibrous grass is relatively low.

Vitamins

Although vitamin A is inefficiently converted from carotene by horses, deficiency is not likely to occur unless grazing is on parched ground where grass is bleached. Occasionally deficiency occurs where housed horses are fed a cereal-based diet and bleached hay.

B vitamins are theoretically manufactured by bacteria in the gut, but there is evidence that young and rapidly growing horses may need a supplement of vitamin B12 in the diet. All horses require vitamin B1 (thiamine) in their diet, although only when thiamine is destroyed in bracken poisoning is a problem likely to occur. Horses kept housed, fed on hay and a high level of oats (that is, horses in training) and lactating mares may develop an anaemia which is characteristic of folic acid deficiency.

There is an interaction between the activity of vitamin E and selenium, so deficiency of either will cause similar signs. Although white muscle disease is recognised in foals whose dams are deficient in vitamin E or selenium, failure of muscle function in adults working physically hard has not been demonstrated. Controversy also exists over whether vitamin E or selenium deficiency is implicated as a contributor to azoturia.

Minerals

Calcium and phosphorus are the two minerals most commonly causing dietary problems. Both are important in bone growth and the two interact. Cereals are naturally low in calcium but contain phosphorus as a phytic acid salt which combines with calcium, preventing it from being absorbed and increasing calcium loss in the faeces. Due to their sites of absorption in the gut, excessive calcium intake has little effect on phosphorus absorption, whereas excessive phosphorus seriously depresses calcium absorption. Hard grasses and hard hay have inadequate calcium levels, whereas wheat bran has a very high phosphorus level. Consequently, this combination leads to a severe calcium deficiency and poor bone formation.

Too rapid growth in the foal is generally considered undesirable as this can lead to abnormalities at the growth plates (the areas near the ends of bones where growth occurs). The problem is further compounded, since poor roughage in the diet can result in phosphorus deficiency which can lead to rickets. In addition, although vitamin D is helpful in the intestine to increase calcium uptake and raise calcium levels in the blood, excessive vitamin D can result in calcium being taken up from the bones, causing thinning of the bones. Supplementation with ground limestone is cheap and likely to prove beneficial.

Sodium, chloride and potassium are minerals which normally occur in abundance in the body. Under certain circumstances, however, deficiencies can arise. In diarrhoea, for example, the normal reabsorption of sodium, potassium and chloride from the intestine is not completed, so that supplementation may be required. After heavy sweating high levels of these three minerals may be lost. This is exacerbated by the fact that the increased energy demand is met by an increase in the cereal component of the diet and a reduction in hay, which results in a fall in the mineral intake. However, forage contains a vast excess of potassium, so only sodium and chloride are normally required. It is likely that deficiencies of these minerals will prove to be far more important than has hitherto been considered possible.

Dietary Allergies

Allergy to certain protein components in the feed is peculiar to some horses. Most frequently it is manifested as small, fluid-filled lumps within the skin, but the lungs may also become involved. By experimenting with the diet and removing the offending food substance, the condition can be spontaneously resolved.

INTESTINAL PARASITES

Many horse owners worm their horses three or four times a year and live happily under the misconception that their protégé is free of parasites until he starts to lose weight inexplicably, or, worse still, has episodes of spasmodic colic. All grazing animals acquire a mixed infection of worms early in life. Severity of the clinical disease resulting from worms merely depends on the burden of worms that is present. In taking appropriate action, the aim is to control the level of infestation since there is no hope of totally eliminating parasites.

Infestations in Foals

Foals start to pick up worms from the first day that they go out on to pasture and, in fact, even before that.

Strongyloides westeri This is a very small worm which usually affects foals of between one and four months. After six months old it is rarely found. It lives in the small intestine and is commonly the cause of diarrhoea in the four- to six-week-old foal. The source of infection is larvae in the dam's milk although larvae can also penetrate through the skin. Mares hold a reservoir of larvae in their tissues. In late pregnancy or early lactation the larvae move to the udder. Treatment of foals is rapidly effective but treatment of the dam to remove the source has little effect.

Parascaris equorum By three months of age a much larger worm up to 50cm in length becomes established in the small intestine. This worm is *Parascaris equorum*. The egg, containing an infective larva, has a very thick protective coat, so that it can survive several years of severe weather conditions. The egg is sticky and easily fastens itself to the passing foal. Eggs are eaten with pasture, and from the intestine the larvae move through the liver to the lungs, where they may cause coughing and a discharge from the nose.

The larvae are coughed up, swallowed again and pass back into the intestine where they become adult and produce eggs themselves.

This prepatent period, as it is called, lasts three months, so infection with adult worms does not occur under three months of age. As the foal becomes adult it may develop an immunity to the worms. The heavy worm burden usually causes unthriftiness and some mild respiratory signs, but occasionally worms can build up in such quantities that they cause a blockage, or even rupture the intestine.

To reduce these worms, foals should be treated monthly after four to eight weeks of age up to six months. Most modern preparations claim to kill ascarids, but the older piperazine is probably still one of the most efficient preparations on the market.

Strongyles

By far the most important intestinal parasites are those living in the caecum and the large intestine – the strongyles. Various species occur, from 1cm to 5cm in size. They are reddish black in colour, and include the most common redworm or bloodworm (*Strongylus vulgaris*) together with the less important but larger *Strongylus edentatus* and *Strongylus equinus*.

S. vulgaris has a prepatent period of six months so does not occur as an adult worm in young foals. It has a complicated life cycle in which larvae are eaten from the pasture and pass to the small intestine. Here they burrow through the intestinal wall and migrate along the tiny arteries which supply the gut, towards a site from which these arteries all disperse towards the gut after leaving the main artery – the aorta. During their migration they cause clots to form in the arteries so that blood, and therefore oxygen, is withheld from the gut. This can be extremely painful and can cause short bouts of colic until a separate blood supply is established. This sort of damage is

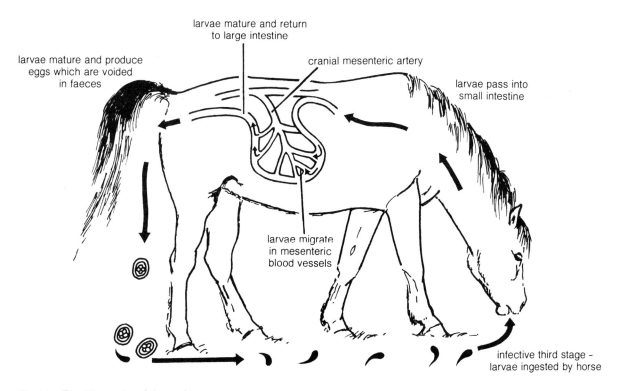

larvae mature and return to large intestine

larvae mature and produce eggs which are voided in faeces

cranial mesenteric artery

larvae pass into small intestine

larvae migrate in mesenteric blood vessels

infective third stage – larvae ingested by horse

Fig 11   The life-cycle of the redworm.

particularly common in horses between a year and three years of age, after which they appear to develop a degree of resistance to the worms.

After three to four months developing in the cranial mesenteric artery (*see Fig 11*), they migrate back to the small intestine, then pass to the large intestine. During the next six weeks or so they mature and start to produce eggs themselves. The adults injure the walls of the colon, damaging blood vessels and causing haemorrhages. This may result in gradual loss of condition and sometimes anaemia. Occasionally they may cause diarrhoea.

Eggs remain inactive over winter on the pasture until the environmental temperature starts to increase. The eggs do not die on the pasture unless the environmental conditions are particularly harsh. When conditions are right, many millions of eggs hatch together, which explains the sudden increase in disease attributable to worms in the spring.

A smaller strongyle – *Trichonema* – does not migrate but lives in the same site. Larvae develop in the intestinal wall. In late winter and early spring there can be a massive emergence of larvae. This may trigger acute diarrhoea which is frequently fatal.

Pinworm

One other common intestinal worm, particularly in young horses, is the pinworm – *Oxyuris equi*. This is significant only in that it lays its eggs around the anus, causing intense irritation which may lead to rubbing at the base of the tail. On close examination, masses of eggs are seen as greyish yellow streaks.

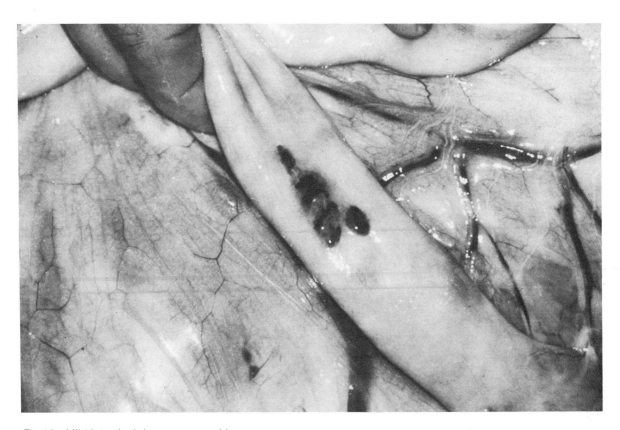

Fig 12   Mild intestinal damage caused by worms.

Bots

Bots are not worms at all, but the larvae of a fly. The adult fly – *Gastrophilus* – can cause annoyance to the horse as it approaches. It lays a mass of yellow eggs on the coat from July to September. The eggs are licked off and pass to the stomach where they remain over winter. In spring, they move through the gut and on to the pasture where they develop into adults. Their significance in the stomach is not fully understood but, using an appropriate preparation in late autumn or winter, they can easily be removed and may be voided in huge numbers, appearing as barrel-shaped, reddish-brown segmented larvae approximately 1cm in length.

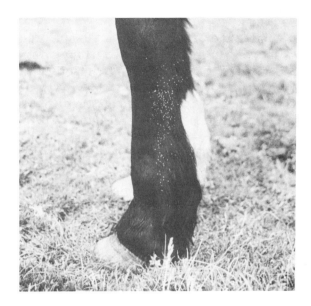

Fig 13 Bot eggs are common in late summer, particularly on the legs.

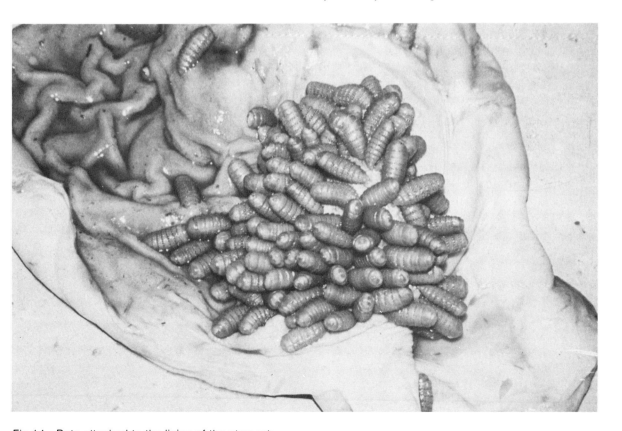

Fig 14 Bots attached to the lining of the stomach.

Tapeworms

Tapeworms occur occasionally in horses following the eating of forage mites which carry the eggs. They occur in the small intestine and caecum and may reach 5cm in length, but they are not considered important and treatment is rare.

Diagnosing Worm Problems

It is often difficult to diagnose when worms are causing disease, since most problems are caused by migrating larvae. Examination of faeces for adult worms is unlikely to be helpful. Even microscopic examination for worm eggs can have very variable results, particularly since the output of eggs varies significantly according to the time of day. Presence of eggs will give a good indication of the presence of adults, but is unlikely to give accurate information on the quantity.

If we look at blood, anaemia may indicate presence of worms, but it may also result from other completely different conditions. Certain white blood cells are increased in response to parasites, which may be helpful, but they are also increased in an allergic response. Perhaps the most useful guide is to look at blood proteins. Certain fractions increase in response to parasites, giving a fairly characteristic distribution pattern, and this is probably the most helpful guide currently available.

Controlling Infestations

A variety of methods can be used to control worms in the horse. Dosing with anthelmintics, the drug used to kill worms, is effective. It is essential to treat all the horses in a given area together, since any not treated will continue to contaminate the pasture. Treatment should be repeated every four to six weeks although during the winter this period can be extended. If possible horses should be put on to clean pasture 24 hours after worming. Any new arrivals should be wormed and isolated for 72 hours before joining the others.

Most anthelmintics available kill only adult strongyles, so the harmful larvae are untouched. Fenbendazole (Panacur), for example, must be given at eight times the normal dose rate to eliminate larvae. Different anthelmintics vary in their effectiveness on different species of worms. *Fig 15* is a table of the preparations currently available.

Several preparations have similar active agents in them. It is fairly common for worms to build up resistance to the active ingredient, necessitating a change to a different drug. If this is the case, a completely different group of drugs must be used, since cross resistance will occur within the groups. A good regime is to use one drug throughout the year until the autumn, then change to one that kills worms and bots, once or twice over winter, before changing to a third type for the next year and returning to the boticide for the winter again.

In addition, good pasture management can be very helpful. If dung is removed from the pasture, levels of infestation are well controlled providing that the dung is removed within 24 hours. After this, larvae will have moved away from the dung on to the pasture.

Where possible, the use of cattle or sheep on the pasture, in rotation with horses, enables them to digest the horse worm eggs and larvae without deleterious effect.

ALIMENTARY TRACT DISORDERS

Choke

The oesophagus or gullet is a long and relatively narrow tube from the mouth to stomach, but it has fairly elastic walls and can be dilated to a degree by passing food. Where the gullet passes from the base of the neck to cross the chest, however, its ability to dilate is limited. Certain feed materials, when eaten

ACTIVITY			DRUG	TRADE NAME	FORMS
adult strongyles	migrating strongyles	bots			
			Pyrantel	Strongid P (Pfizer)	Paste, granules
			Thiaben-dazole	Equizole (MSD) Thibenzole (MSD)	Paste, powder Paste, pellets, powder
			Oxiben-dazole	Equitac (Smith Kline) Lincoln horse & pony wormer (Battle, Hayward & Bower) Rycovet horse & pony wormer (Rycovet)	Paste Paste Paste
			Mebenda-zole	Equiverm Plus (Crown) Telmin (Crown)	Paste, powder Paste
			Febantel	Bayverm (Bayer)	Paste, pellets
			Fenbenda-zole	Panacur (Hoechst)	Paste, suspension, powder, granules
			Oxfenda-zole	Synanthic (Syntex) Systamex (Coopers)	Paste, pellets Paste
			Ivermectin	Eqvalan (MSS)	Paste
			Dichlorvos	Astrobot (Arnolds) Frisk (Pettifer)	Granules Granules
			Haloxon	Equilox (Crown)	Paste
			Metripho-nate	Bayverm Plus (Bayer) Neguvon (Bayer)	Paste Paste

Note: Horizontal lines separate chemical groups. When changing to avoid a build-up of resistance, change between groups. Broken lines indicate variable activity at normal recommended rates.

Fig 15 Currently available worming preparations, showing spectrum of activity and available forms.

rapidly and not properly chewed, can become lodged in the oesophagus. Large pieces of carrot are the most common feedstuffs to do this. Often though, the choke results from the eating of a dried feed which swells as it becomes wet. Sugar beet does this most frequently, although horse or pony nuts can produce the same effect. As they are mixed with saliva, they swell enormously and become wedged in the oesophagus. By the time the horse realises that it has a problem, food may have accumulated over a considerable length of the oesophagus. For this reason, sugar beet must be soaked for twelve hours before it is fed, to allow it to absorb water and to swell.

The choked horse is not in immediate danger but becomes very distressed. Saliva continues to be produced but, being unable to reach the stomach, fills the oesophagus before overflowing back from the mouth and nose. The horse stands with neck extended and coughs saliva. At this point there is a danger that saliva will be inhaled and establish a pneumonia. Veterinary attention is urgently required, if only to relax the horse. Meanwhile, all sources of food and bedding should be removed to prevent further eating which may compound the problem. It is desirable to make the horse relax as much as possible which will allow the oesophagus to dilate. This can be helped by leaving the horse alone and in an unstimulated state. If necessary, a tranquilliser can be given to achieve relaxation. The veterinary surgeon may also attempt to move the food material, using a nasogastric tube introduced into the oesophagus through the nose. Gentle pushing may dislodge an obstruction but, failing this, small quantities of water passed down and then sucked out again may remove the obstruction a little at a time. Clearance of the oesophagus may require several attempts over two or three days, but the obstruction nearly always clears successfully eventually without recourse to surgery.

Colic

The term 'colic' is somewhat emotive but simply means abdominal pain, although it is usually confined to abdominal pain originating in the alimentary tract. It is essential, however, to establish from the outset that the pain does result from abnormality in the gut rather than, say, a gynaecological problem in the pregnant mare, testicular pain in the stallion or even laminitis or rupture of the diaphragm separating the abdomen from the chest. Horses with these conditions share many of the symptoms associated with colic.

In the early stages, the horse may simply look dull and miserable, looking round occasionally at his flanks and pawing the ground. There may be bouts of patchy sweating. As the condition progresses, the sweating may become more profuse. The abdomen may be distended and the horse may kick periodically at it. The respiratory rate may increase a little and the heart rate also rises. Finally, the horse may start to roll, to walk backwards or to adopt a position resembling a sitting dog. The healthy pink of the mucous membranes around the eye gives way to a darker red, and in prolonged cases may take on a yellow tinge. When the signs are mild, it is as well to observe the horse for an hour or so. Frequently the symptoms will pass. If they do not recur over the next two hours, it is safe to assume that all is well. If the signs do not pass, or become more severe, veterinary help should be summoned urgently. When the signs are severe, help should be requested immediately, although this should be done without panic.

Colic is not a disease, and a diagnosis still needs to be made. The causes of colic are many, so the administration of a 'colic drench' is unlikely to be beneficial, since the cause of the pain has first to be established. A 'colic drench' can only be helpful if it relieves pain, which it is unlikely to do effectively. Even if it does, it may then complicate the picture for any attending veterinary surgeon. Furthermore, there is a good chance that some of the drench will be inhaled, resulting in a pneumonia to compound the problems. The drench may even do exactly the opposite of what is required. If treatment is needed, it is better left to the veterinary surgeon.

While waiting for a veterinary surgeon, it is best to remove any food and water. Gentle walking is probably helpful, as it allows the horse to feel more comfortable. Movement often increases gut activity, so that material is passed on through as much as possible. It may also prevent the horse from rolling and injuring himself in the process. He should not, however, be forced to walk when he is exhausted and in this state he should be allowed to lie down. It is a common misconception that horses who roll will 'twist their gut'. If the gut does twist during rolling, there is a high probability that it would have done so if the horse had remained standing. Horses with a normal gut do not twist it when rolling.

Several bodily processes go wrong in the most common type of colic, spasmodic colic, in which the horse may show periods of intense pain lasting from a few minutes up to an hour or more.

Food is moved along the intestine by peristalsis in which a wave of muscle contractions in the intestinal wall moves along the length of the intestine behind the food, pushing the food in front of it, away from the mouth. In addition, contractions of segments of intestine and random churnings help to aid movement. These movements require sodium and oxygen. Consequently, under certain circumstances when inadequate sodium is supplied, horses will show signs of abdominal pain and muscle cramps in the abdomen. This may happen where salt is not supplied in the diet and where high levels of sodium are lost in sweating. The oxygen supply to a length of gut can also be stopped if there is damage to the blood vessels supplying that area. Most frequently damage results from the activity of redworm larvae which migrate along the

blood vessel walls during larval development. Again the horse will show signs of intense abdominal pain.

Once the movement in the gut stops, natural gas production causes stretching of the intestinal walls. The stretched muscle of the walls becomes less efficient at contracting, even when oxygen is supplied, and the problem compounds. The abdomen is not an empty, barrel-like structure with a few loops of intestine suspended in the middle of it; it is an outer skin, packed with intestines and other organs, and there is no space whatsoever between loops of gut. Usually the affected piece of gut establishes an alternative blood supply, oxygen is replaced and the colic subsides. Sometimes, however, when large areas of gut are affected, much gas is allowed to build up. The gut then resembles a balloon under water – it becomes unstable, rides up through the other intestines and can easily flip over, causing a twist which makes it resemble a sausage. Alternatively, and more commonly, it can rotate on the tissue which suspends it from the area below the spine and in which the blood supply runs. When this happens the blood supply to the whole length of intestine can be strangled.

Since the initial damage frequently results from worm infestation, this type of colic is most frequently seen in spring and autumn when worm activity is at its greatest. It is also more common in young horses and it is probable that older horses develop a degree of resistance to redworms.

Assessing the condition Although horses are very susceptible to pain and it is therefore essential to control the pain level as rapidly as possible, this should not be done until the state of the horse has been fully assessed. More important than the state of the horse when first examined is how that state is changing. This means that the condition must be monitored constantly using certain criteria.

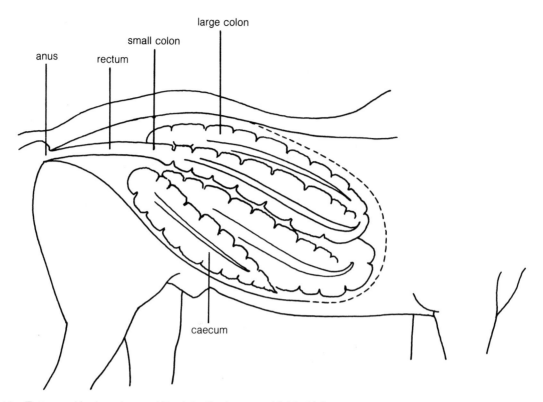

Fig 16   Topographical anatomy of the intestinal organs (right side).

A low pulse which is rapidly rising, for example, is more worrying than a higher pulse that is static or falling. Much can be learned by listening to the gut activity, but more can be gained by feeling the state of the intestines through the wall of the rectum with a hand carefully introduced into the rectum. This is a potentially hazardous procedure since the rectum can easily tear. The introduction of a tube through the nose into the stomach can give valuable information, as can the introduction of a needle through the wall of the abdomen to draw fluid from around the intestines. The appearance of any fluid thus obtained can be extremely helpful. A blood sample taken in the early stages of colic can be useful to provide a baseline in assessing the state of shock which will inevitably occur. Again, it can be compared against subsequent samples to assess the rate of deterioration.

Fortunately the vast majority of colics can be resolved with simple medical treatment.

Tympanitic colic   Also known as flatulent colic, this is characterised by a build-up of gas due to the excessive fermentation of lush foods such as clover, grass cuttings or apples. The abdomen is distended and tense and the pain is severe. When distended, the wall of the intestine frequently goes into spasm, and a spasmolytic drug is often beneficial in reducing this spasm. Although this state usually resolves quickly with treatment, the condition can make the horse particularly susceptible to a subsequent twisting of the gut. The likelihood of twisting is greater due to increased activity in the gut and the horse often finishes the colic with diarrhoea.

Impaction Low grade pain over a prolonged period is the characteristic of an impaction in the gut, usually at the pelvic flexure (bend) as previously described. In the early stages, normal dung is passed until all contents beyond the site of obstruction are voided, then the level drops to dry, scanty faeces or even none at all. The causes of impaction are numerous. It may result from eating poor quality roughage such as straw, or better quality roughage which has not been properly chewed because the teeth require attention. Restricted access to water may be a cause, as may injury to the wall of the colon as a result of redworm damage.

Affected horses are seldom in great pain and it is often sufficient to give purgatives: mineral oil, such as medicinal liquid paraffin, which slightly irritates the gut lining, increasing activity and lubricating the contents, or saline, which draws water into the gut from the blood so softening the contents. If the condition continues for more than two to three days, however, complications may arise as a result of starvation.

Where the colic is mild the horse will benefit from being allowed water. Once the impaction has cleared, food should be gradually reintroduced.

Obstruction Occasionally the gut becomes completely obstructed, either from material inside which cannot be moved on, or from material becoming wrapped around the segment, which, again, cannot be removed. A further possibility, where there has been intense activity, is that one segment of gut has telescoped into the next, causing a blockage. All these situations will show more severe signs than those previously mentioned, and they will clearly not respond to medical treatment. With time they will become more serious until, without surgical intervention, they will prove fatal.

Once the parameters of the condition have reached the point where surgery becomes inevitable, it is necessary to decide whether it should be attempted. If it is agreed that this line should not be taken, it is only humane to destroy the horse. If surgery is undertaken quickly, that is, within approximately eight hours of the start of the process which has rendered surgery necessary, the prospect of a satisfactory outcome is frequently good.

Diarrhoea

Transient, self-limiting diarrhoea may result from sudden changes in diet, excitement or transport and provided that faecal consistency returns to normal within two or three days, it is of little consequence. All other episodes of diarrhoea are potentially very serious and frequently prove fatal.

Nutritional factors are often responsible for diarrhoea, especially where feedstuffs such as grass clippings or barley, which are highly prone to fermentation, are fed. Once the offending material has passed through the intestine, the diarrhoea is likely to cease.

With the introduction of modern anthelmintics, the use of 'physics' such as anthraquinone or aloes to worm horses has gone out of fashion. These substances acted by causing excessive movement in the intestine, often together with colic. When this treatment was overdone, a severe diarrhoea was produced.

Some antibiotics which act against a wide spectrum of bacteria can also cause diarrhoea if given by mouth. The level of some antibiotics in bile, and hence in the intestines, is five to ten times that found in the blood. The antibiotics kill the large number of normal bacteria present, particularly in the colon and caecum, which are essential for normal digestion. Consequently the way is left clear for many dangerous (pathogenic) bacteria and fungi to multiply, resulting in a superinfection which can be extremely difficult to overcome.

Perhaps the most important group of bacteria to take advantage of this situation is the *salmonellae* which take many forms or serotypes (sub-types). The severity of symptoms which they produce can be wide ranging. Up to 2 per cent of normal horses shed salmonellae in their faeces and up to 12.5 per cent may be carriers, showing no signs of the disease. When stressed, for example by being transported, anaesthetised, starved or wormed, or treated with certain antibiotics, horses release a potent cellular poison (endotoxin) over the next four days, which damages the gut lining and causes a shock-like syndrome. Fever, colic and loss of appetite all accompany a watery, foul-smelling diarrhoea which may contain blood. This rapidly leads to dehydration and loss of some essential minerals and proteins from the body.

A similar syndrome, or collection of symptoms, which is often more severe and rapidly fatal is known as colitis X, 'X' referring to the unknown cause. Again the signs are those of shock produced by endotoxins which may be triggered by stress factors. A high body temperature rapidly falls to below normal, the horse's extremities become cold and death occurs after between three and twenty-four hours.

Infection inside the abdomen, either from a penetrating wound or from an abscess in the gut wall which may burst, produces signs of colic and watery diarrhoea up to a week after the initial introduction of infection.

Other poisons within the intestine can also cause diarrhoea, the most notable being castor beans, organophosphorus insecticides, potatoes and rhododendron, the latter usually producing much salivation and being probably the only substance likely to cause vomiting in the horse.

Treatment In all these cases of diarrhoea the mortality rate is high. Treatment must be given early to be successful and is expensive and time consuming. The most important aspect of treatment in acute cases is the giving of fluids, to prevent shock, directly into the blood, since the ability to absorb fluids from the gut is lost. Tens of litres of fluid are re-

quired to be effective. When chronic diarrhoea is being treated, fluids are not required since the system adjusts to its increased fluid loss. Since, in these cases, time is less critical, a better attempt can be made to establish the cause of the diarrhoea and specific treatment can be given. The damage will often resolve spontaneously if supportive treatment can be given in the meantime, but this may take several months. The aim is to maintain or even increase the scouring horse's bodyweight. Nevertheless, 35 per cent of chronically scouring horses are destroyed.

Establishing causes In trying to establish the cause of chronic diarrhoea, your veterinary surgeon will require details of recent diet and changes in diet, how much your horse is eating and drinking and whether he has developed abnormal preferences. It is also helpful for him to know what measures have been taken to control parasites, whether any stressful incidents have recently occurred, whether any weight loss started before or after the onset of diarrhoea and whether any other horses are similarly affected. He will also want to make a detailed clinical examination, probably involving laboratory assessment of parasites or bacteria in the faeces, and an examination of blood. This will help him to assess dehydration, changes in the white blood cells indicating infections or some types of tumours and biochemical factors which may point to damage in the liver.

Once again, worms are most likely to be the cause, particularly in the spring, in horses who have shown poor condition in the winter. These horses respond reasonably well to treatment that includes anthelmintics to kill the worm larvae.

Chronic salmonella infection leads to diarrhoea characterised by emaciation and recurrent bouts of colic. In these cases, as in those where forms of neoplasia (tumours) affect the intestine, prospects of recovery are not good.

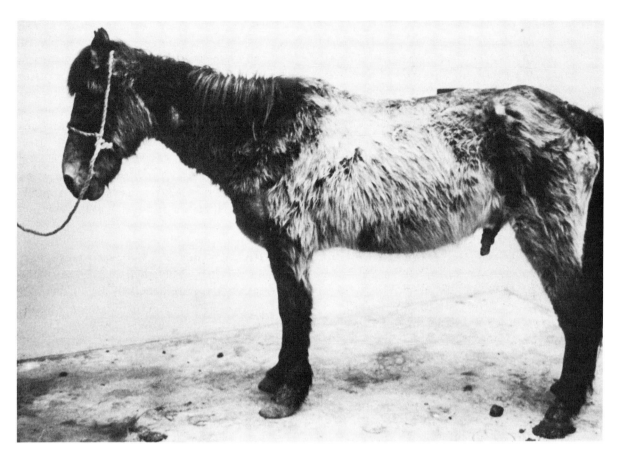

Fig 17   Emaciation as a result of chronic diarrhoea, probably caused by worm damage.

The Thin Horse

Often when a horse is losing weight the cause is obvious – he has been deprived of food, he has suffered from a prolonged period of diarrhoea or he has not been wormed recently. However, sometimes the cause is not immediately clear. In these cases we must decide whether the horse seems well, apart from the weight loss, or not.

The healthy horse   If he does appear well, we should carefully consider whether an adequate quantity of food, of the right type, is being fed, whether he is actually eating it, and not being bullied by others, and whether the food is being properly digested. Have his teeth checked. Also check that fresh, clean water is always available. Look at his exercise routine. Horses do not respond well to long periods of exercise at weekends if they do nothing during the week, so exercise should be as regular as possible. If all seems correct, the worming position should be re-checked.

Finally, some older horses seem unable to cope adequately with anything but grass, so over winter they may lose weight while still eating adequate hay and concentrates. As soon as they are turned back on to spring grass they put on weight again. The best treatment for these animals is to try to find grazing which is adequate to last through the winter.

Certain vitamin deficiencies can cause weight loss. Folic acid, one of the B group, causes a characteristic anaemia in Thoroughbreds and halfbreds which are kept housed and fed on hay. It is easily corrected by dietary supplementation.

The sick horse Where the horse is unwell, the cause of weight loss is often easier to ascertain. Continual low-grade pain, such as a chronic lameness, may have this effect.

The horse may have lost his ability to swallow. This may be very slight and difficult to see. The horse may eat slowly and clumsily – the difficulty is more obvious when drinking is attempted. Such signs may follow a chronic upper respiratory tract infection, chronic grass disease, botulism after eating bagged silage, or lead poisoning. (For further information, *see* Chapter 11.)

Chronic conditions, particularly suppurating infections, often result in a loss of condition. Chronic liver disease means that the liver does not produce the proteins required to build up the tissues. Chronic kidney disease, although rare, may result in proteins being lost in the urine. Abnormalities of the heart are quite common, but rarely cause the horse to lose weight unless the heart deteriorates in condition after exercise.

Vices are often responsible for a horse being thin, most notably excessive crib biting and wind sucking, and mares with excessive sexual activity may lose weight.

Finally, the skin should be carefully checked in the thin horse. A heavy louse infestation causes a marked loss in flesh, and continual rubbing of a skin irritation may reduce the time spent eating.

Where the cause of weight loss is not obvious, it may take several hard looks to reach a conclusion, backed by a battery of laboratory tests which can be very expensive.

The Liver

Structure and physiology The horse's liver weighs approximately 5kg and occupies the front of the abdomen adjacent to the diaphragm, predominantly on the right side. It is the largest gland in the body and in draught horses it may weigh 8-9kg, receiving most products absorbed from the small intestine into the portal system. The portal system consists of any vein which collects blood from one network of capillaries (tiny enmeshed blood vessels) and carries it directly to a second network of capillaries in another part of the body without first returning it to the heart. In the case of the liver, it is the hepatic portal vein that carries blood containing the absorbed products of digestion from the intestine directly to the liver.

Many of the liver's functions relate to the metabolism or processing of these products from the small intestine. The liver plays a key role in the formation of glucose from stored forms (glycogen), lactate from muscle and amino acids from protein breakdown. The lower fatty acids (propionic, acetic and butyric acids) which are produced in the caecum and colon are metabolised here. Some glycogen is stored in the liver, and acts as a limited source of glucose. During starvation glucose is derived from protein breakdown. Proteins cannot be stored in the body, so protein breakdown and the formation of new proteins is important.

Fats are made in the liver from carbohydrates and broken down protein. Breakdown products of fats are supplied from the digestive tract. The liver controls the storage depots for fats, both in the liver and elsewhere. Transport of fat from the liver relies on a good provision of B vitamins and these need to be supplied when the liver is damaged.

The liver is important in producing bile to dissolve and absorb dietary fat. Bile also removes cholesterol and some of the breakdown products of blood. Destruction of red blood cells is another function of the liver. Bile is continuously formed in large quantities.

Many of the harmful waste products and other absorbed materials are detoxified by the liver, rendering them harmless before removal from the body. When the liver is damaged, toxic products may accumulate.

Two further functions of the liver are the formation of blood proteins and the storage of vitamins. It can be readily appreciated, therefore, that diseases involving the liver produce symptoms involving a wide range of systems, reflecting the importance of this organ. Similarly, treatment of liver disease requires attention to many factors which may become affected by the pathological process.

Liver disease 75 per cent of the functional capacity of the liver must be lost before clinical signs of disease become apparent, and then the onset of disease in acute or chronic states is sudden.

Acute liver disease is very severe and dangerous, occurring in summer and autumn, since it usually results from the eating of toxic substances in one of more than a hundred suitable varieties of pasture plants, or from certain chemical toxins – arsenic, lead, copper, phosphorus, nitrite and carbon tetrachloride.

The signs exhibited are of depression, with the eyes partially closed, head drooping and yawning. Hay may remain part chewed, in the mouth. The horse walks compulsively but appears blind. Nervous signs appear because ammonia produced in the intestine is not removed by the damaged liver in the normal fashion. Ammonia damages nerves and so has greatest effect on the brain. In addition, the amount of glucose released by the liver into the blood is reduced. Since the brain is the organ most reliant on glucose to function, it suffers the greatest effect from shortage.

After 24 to 48 hours, jaundice may develop. This may be the result of increased production of pigment due to the breakdown of red blood cells, or more usually to a reduction in the rate

of removal of pigment, either as a result of damage to the liver cells, or obstruction of the ducts down which the bile flows to leave the liver. The urine may also be dark, since some pigment is lost by this route. Reduction of bile flow often leads to constipation and vague abdominal discomfort. In the later stages of liver disease a staggering gait may develop, the head may be pressed against a wall or hard surface, the horse may become excited and go into convulsions, coma and death.

Where recovery does occur, laminitis may follow, which suggests a toxic cause of laminitis.

Another sequel to liver disease is photosensitization. Normally chlorophyll, the green pigment of plants, is broken down by bacteria in the gut into phylloerythrin which is subsequently removed by the liver and passed out in bile. When the liver is damaged, phylloerythrin is passed into the blood and circulates. In areas of skin where there is no pigment to protect it – either white areas or flesh marks – the phylloerythrin absorbs the ultraviolet sunlight, causing it to damage the adjacent tissues. As a result, severe inflammation develops in these areas.

Chronic liver disease is insidious in its onset. It shows first as weight loss, lack of appetite, a slight instability in the gait, constipation and sometimes a fluid swelling under the skin along the belly. As in the acute (sudden) form, there may be yawning, pressing of the head and food left in the mouth, but jaundice is slight or absent.

The chronic (longer lasting) disease is more common than the acute form and may be a low grade response to the chemical or plant toxins which produce the acute form. More frequently, however, it results from eating plants of the genus *Senecio*, namely ragwort or groundsel or *Equisetum* (horsetails). These plants are bitter so are not usually eaten when green, but are palatable in hay. They cause cirrhosis of the liver cells – a process in which the cells become fibrous and which is irreversible.

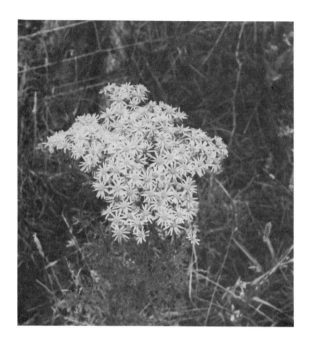

Fig 18   Ragwort, which causes irreversible liver damage to the horse.

Liver damage can occasionally be caused by the formation of a chronic abscess, and liver fluke (parasitic flatworm) infestation has been recorded in horses. Liver fluke, bots or ascarid worms may invade and block the bile duct, causing an obstructive jaundice. Confirmation of liver disease is by biochemical examination of blood samples and examination of a small sample of liver (a biopsy).

Hyperlipaemia is a condition, generally occurring in fat ponies, which resembles liver disease in clinical signs. It results from a sudden carbohydrate deficit which may be caused by complete starvation, as occurs when treatment of ponies with laminitis is too enthusiastic, or in late pregnancy when feed intake is inadequate. The pony's response is to mobilise his fat reserves, pouring fat into the blood and choking the liver. Immediate treatment is needed to remove the fat, since the condition is rapidly fatal.

5 Respiratory System

The definition of the word 'respire' is 'to breathe in and out'. Why does the horse need to breathe in and out and how does he do so?

FUNCTIONS OF RESPIRATION

In order to survive, the horse needs energy; energy to keep warm, energy to enable his heart to beat and energy to move his limbs. The digestive system supplies the fuel to provide that energy, as food which is then converted by the digestive tract and liver into fats, carbohydrates and protein – the fuels. In order to burn these fuels, thus supplying energy, the body needs oxygen. While the fuels are burning, waste products are produced which have to be eliminated from the body before they cause any harm. The main functions of the respiratory tract are, therefore, first to transport air into the body, where the oxygen can be absorbed into the system, and second to get rid of some of the waste products that form during energy production. The gas carbon dioxide and excess heat are two of the most important waste products that the respiratory system removes from the body.

STRUCTURE OF THE RESPIRATORY SYSTEM

In order to carry out its functions, the respiratory system has developed a complicated series of tubes and chambers which carry the air into and out of the body, and an arrangement of bones and muscles which, acting rather like bellows, first expand to suck the air in, then contract to force the air out.

Nose and Throat

The passage of the air through this arrangement of tubes starts at the two nostrils. From here, the air moves along the nose, past a series of bony plates called the turbinates, to the back of the throat. The surfaces of the turbinates are covered with a lining, the mucous membrane, which secretes a sticky fluid called mucus. The membrane and the mucus together act as a barrier to foreign material. The membrane, with its good blood supply, warms the air and the mucus traps some of the dust particles.

The sinuses, both frontal and maxillary, open into this passage, as do two more sacs called the guttural pouches. The exact physiological function of these cavities is not clear, but from the veterinary point of view they are important because they are occasionally the site of disease.

The warmed and washed air now passes through the pharynx – the chamber at the back of the throat – into the voice box, larynx, and down the windpipe, trachea, into the chest.

Chest

Soon after the trachea enters the chest, it divides into two tubes, the left and right bronchi. Further subdivisions occur, into medium-sized and then smaller tubes called bronchioles. Each bronchiole ends in small air sacs called alveoli. The whole structure can be likened to an inverted tree, with the trunk as the trachea, the branches the bronchi, twigs the bronchioles and leaves the alveoli.

Alveoli It is here that the real work of the respiratory system takes place. Through the wall of the alveoli, a process called gaseous

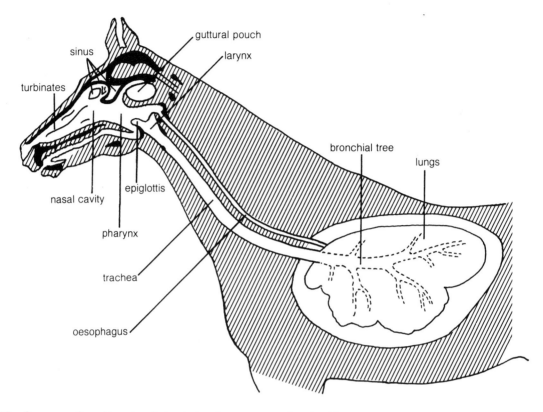

Fig 19   Cross-section of head and chest, showing component parts of the respiratory system.

exchange occurs. Each alveolus has a fine network of small blood vessels surrounding it. The proximity of the blood vessels, and the single cell layer of the alveolus wall, allow molecules of oxygen to squeeze through into the capillary blood vessel. One of the waste products of metabolism, carbon dioxide, passes the other way, from capillary blood vessel into the alveolus and from there is removed from the body as the horse breathes out.

Muscles The work necessary to move such large volumes of air in and out of the horse's lungs is done mainly by the muscles of the chest and diaphragm. When respiratory effort is great, after hard work or when breathing is difficult due to disease, the muscles of the abdomen play an increasing part in the respira-

tory cycle. The muscles which do much of the work of breathing are called the intercostal muscles. They lie between the ribs and when they contract they lift the walls of the chest up and out, thus increasing the volume of the chest cavity. The lungs, being elastic structures, expand to fill the extra space. Air then rushes in and fills the extra volume created in the lungs. This part of the respiratory cycle is called inspiration.

Breathing out, or expiration, does not take so much work and the elasticity of the lungs helps considerably. The lungs resemble a blown-up balloon; when released, the balloon contracts and the air rushes out. In much the same way, once the intercostal muscles relax, the lungs spring back to their original volume, dragging the chest wall down and in, and forcing air out of the body.

RESPIRATORY DISORDERS

Causes

Having worked out why and how a horse respires, and before we categorise all the diseases that affect his respiratory system, it would be as well to consider why these diseases develop.

Man is the culprit. Man, by selective breeding, has introduced congenital abnormalities (defects normally present at birth, and often inherited), such as a small epiglottis, which adversely affect respiration. By his insistence on housing large numbers of susceptible horses together, man has certainly increased the incidence of infectious disease. We should remember that the horse, in its wild state, is used to living in small groups on vast grassy plains, with plenty of space in which to run, clean air to breathe and few other horses from whom infectious diseases can be caught. The horse's large lungs and his straight airway, free from obstructions, which connects the lungs to outside air, are superbly adapted to ensure that his body always has enough oxygen to keep his fuel burning, allowing him to move.

Noisy Breathing

Is he clean in the wind? This is the first question asked when considering a new purchase. The horse who makes a noise when breathing hard is universally condemned, but need he be?

The first priority is to decide whether the noise occurs when the horse breathes out, or when he breathes both in and out. The first is of little consequence; all horses make a noise when cantering or galloping, and if this noise occurs on expiration, with a few exceptions, it has no effect on performance. The horse who high blows is a good example. This noise is caused by resonance in the false nostril and, in spite of its disconcerting noise, it has no effect on performance.

Roarers, whistlers and noisy horses The whistler or roarer is another matter. Here the noise is caused by a defect in the larynx or pharynx which obstructs the air flow into the lungs. When the horse is in hard work, he needs all the air he can get. Any obstruction will reduce the amount of oxygen reaching his system, with a corresponding reduction in performance.

So far, no single condition that might cause such a noise has been mentioned. All too often it is assumed that the cause of any noise is a paralysed vocal cord, and that the treatment must be a Hobday operation. A more sensible plan would be to examine the area first and find out what is happening. With the help of an endoscope, we can do just that. An endoscope is a wonderful instrument which allows us to see around corners. If it is inserted into the nostril and carefully advanced, the first area to come into view is the nasal chamber. It is here that the first abnormalities which could cause such a noise are found.

ABNORMALITIES OF THE NASAL CHAMBERS

Nasal Polyps and Tumours

Nasal polyps are soft, pedunculated growths (growths attached by a stalk) which are found on the surface of the nasal chamber. The air rushing past the growth quickly damages the surface, which becomes dead. The degenerating areas begin to smell, the breath becomes fetid and bleeding sometimes occurs.

Many other tumours can develop in this area. Generally, by the time they are noticed, they have become so extensive that radical surgery is necessary to remove them and the chance of recovery is not good.

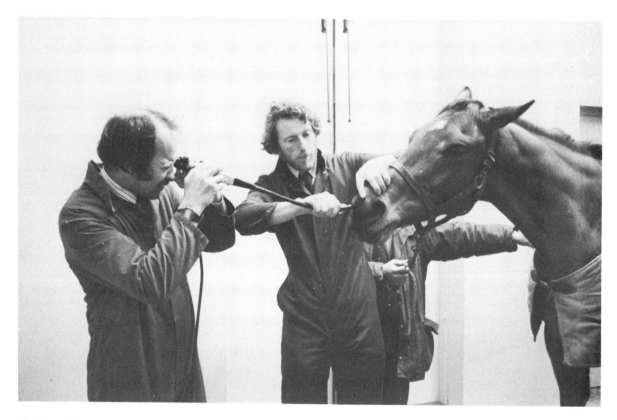

Fig 20   Using an endoscope to examine the respiratory tract.

Sinus Infections

The major sinuses of the head enter into the nasal chamber and can be seen as slit-like openings in the wall.

The sinuses of the horse can, as in the human, become infected. This generally occurs as a complication of a primary respiratory infection. Pus forms in the cavity and can be seen seeping out of the sinus into the nasal cavity, or can be shown visually by an X-ray of the head, when the pus can be seen as a horizontal line of fluid.

Infection of the other pair of sinuses, the guttural pouches, can also occur. These pouches are unique to the horse and lie in the angle of the jaw. They are a natural enlargement of a tube, called the eustachian tube, which joins the middle ear to the pharynx.

Infection of these pouches is potentially serious, as important arteries and nerves lie in the wall and can easily become damaged by such an infection.

Pharyngitis

As the endoscope advances, we can inspect the pharynx and check whether the noisy breathing is caused by a chronic inflammation of the mucous membrane.

Pharyngeal lymphoid hyperplasia is the rather long name which more accurately describes this condition in the horse. It is common in young horses in training and is their reaction to the constant barrage of infection to which they are subjected. Thick plaques of lymphoid tissue develop and can be seen like bunches of grapes in the pharyngeal roof. This tissue is responsible for producing disease-fighting antibodies and lymphocytes, a type of white blood cell. Young children have a similar problem when they first go to school. The treatment, on the rare occasions it is necessary, is to cauterise the wall of the pharynx with acid or heat.

ABNORMALITIES OF THE THROAT

Further on, at the back of the pharynx, we can now view the entrance to the larynx. This is shaped rather like the entrance to a Greek temple; the epiglottis, tongue shaped, is the flight of steps, the vocal cords, one to each side, can be likened to Grecian pillars, and forming the roof are the arytenoid cartilages.

The failure of this entrance to open fully during inspiration is the cause of another condition which leads to an inspiratory noise.

Laryngeal Hemiplegia

Laryngeal hemiplegia or paralysis of the left vocal cord is a condition which the advent of the endoscope proved to be more common than was formerly realised. Indeed, work done in the United States suggests that the incidence of this condition in the Thoroughbred could be as high as 90 per cent.

In the normal horse, the muscles connected to the arytenoid cartilages contract during inspiration, thus pulling the vocal cords up and out and increasing the size of the laryngeal opening. The more forceful the inspiratory effort, the wider the opening. Horses who suffer from laryngeal hemiplegia do not fully abduct the left vocal cord, and the entrance becomes asymmetrical. The resulting turbulent air flow vibrates the vocal cords, causing the whistling or roaring noise characteristic of the condition. As the severity of the condition increases, so does the degree of obstruction, and with less air entering the body the ability

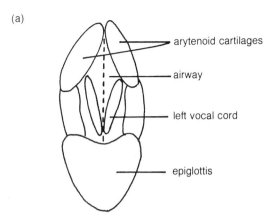

(a)

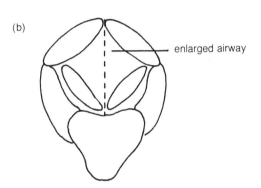

(b)

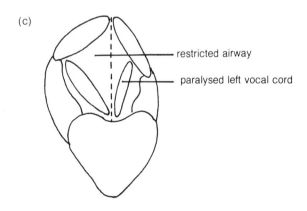

(c)

Fig 21   The larynx under different conditions.

(a) Larynx during quiet respiration at rest.
(b) Larynx during extreme exercise.
(c) Laryngeal paralysis and a restricted airway during fast exercise.

to work is greatly diminished.

The reason for this paralysis is not known. One clue might be the high incidence of paralysis on the left side. The left, recurrent laryngeal nerve which controls the muscle on that side is considerably longer than that on the right, and passes close to the pulsating aorta, a major artery from the heart. The constant beating may damage the nerve, causing a varying degree of paralysis in the muscle.

Surgical interference is the only cure and the traditional method is the Hobday operation. To perform this operation, the larynx is opened. A pouch called the ventricle, which lies behind the vocal cord, is then removed. The theory *was* that the scar tissue, which forms during healing, pulls the vocal cords back and increases the size of the laryngeal opening. Unfortunately, looking at the entrance of the larynx with an endoscope after the operation, when all the tissues have healed, shows that the left vocal cord often remains in the same position as before the operation.

The success of the treatment is difficult to determine as very few horses stop making a noise, although the performance of some does improve. One reason for the improved performance could be the effect of the scar tissue which forms after the operation. Although Hobdaying does not alter the position of the vocal cords, the scar tissue may improve the air flow, making it easier for the horse to breathe. It is also possible that the psychological effect of the operation on the trainer might produce a more suitable training schedule, leading to a fitter horse which, in spite of its disability, is more able to perform.

A more modern method of treatment for this condition is to open the larynx and to tie back the paralysed vocal cord. The technical precision needed to perform this operation does lead to variable results, but when performed successfully, the laryngeal opening is enlarged, allowing free passage of air in and out of the lungs.

The arrangement of the larynx and pharynx relative to each other is also very important. Any alteration of their positions exaggerates an obstruction and makes an already present noise more evident. A horse in a collected canter is much more noisy than when at a free gallop. The angle between neck and head is more acute in the collected canter and the maximum flexion occurs at the pharynx which, as it compresses, obstructs the air flow. At the gallop, the head and neck and enclosed structures are almost in a straight line so when the horse most wants an unimpeded air flow, he gets it.

Soft Palate Dislocation

Sometimes when the horse is at full extension, something goes drastically wrong, and a condition occurs which in racing terms is described as 'swallowing the tongue'. A high-pitched gurgle is suddenly heard, the horse stops, as if hitting a wall and then, after swallowing several times, is able to carry on.

To understand this occurrence, we must first know what happens when a horse swallows. During normal breathing, the larynx sits in the middle of a fold of tissue, rather like a canoeist surrounded by the canoe skirt. When the horse swallows, the larynx is pulled out of the skirt to lie underneath. The entrance of the larynx is closed and any food is directed into the oesophagus by the folds of the pharynx. The larynx then returns to its usual place, allowing breathing to continue.

When the horse 'swallows his tongue' the larynx is stuck under the folds. Any attempt to breathe in pulls the fold over the laryngeal opening, and immediately the horse chokes. Breathing out does not help much, as the folds then vibrate in the pharynx causing a typical gurgling noise. Repeated swallowing eventually returns the larynx to its usual place and breathing resumes as normal. The use of a tongue strap to prevent the larynx from being pulled out of the folds sometimes prevents this condition, but a better method is to cut the

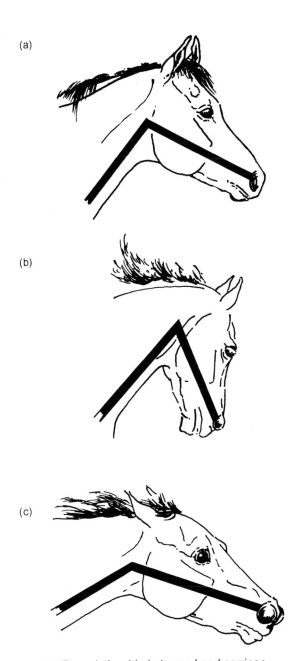

(a)

(b)

(c)

Fig 22 The relationship between head carriage and respiratory noise.

(a) Normal head position.
(b) The more acute angle created during a collected canter leads to an obstructed airway and an increase in noise.
(c) At a full gallop the head and neck are fully extended, the airway is almost straight and offers little resistance to the flow of air.

muscles responsible for displacing the larynx, or to remove part of the folds to lessen the chance of the larynx being trapped.

As we advance through the larynx, we enter the trachea; to reach the bifurcation (branching into two) of the bronchi a long endoscope tube is required, but it is at this level that we see signs of two more important conditions affecting the respiratory system.

ABNORMALITIES OF THE LUNG

Epistaxis (Nose Bleeds)

Some 'bleeders' are evident from blood at the nose, but in many cases we have to reach the trachea before we see signs which tell us that the horse is a nose bleeder. Again, it is the endoscope which enables us to find out exactly where the blood is coming from, and in the vast majority of cases we now know that the lung is the source of the blood.

We know that the posterior tip of the lung is the area most likely to bleed, but not the exact reason why. This area of the lung is subjected to the greatest forces exerted on the lung during breathing and it is possible that during extreme effort, the force is enough to rupture some of the small blood vessels in this area. Any condition likely to increase the forces acting on the lung, such as chronic inflammation of the lung or obstruction of the airway, increases the chance of this occurring.

Haemorrhage can also occur from the upper respiratory tract. However, by the time blood is noticed at the nostrils, the causal lesion is usually quite evident. Nasal polyps and tumours, especially a very vascular tumour called an ethmoid haematoma, all start to bleed as they get larger and their surface becomes more damaged.

A potentially serious haemorrhage is one which originates in the guttural pouch. A large artery runs across the wall of the pouch, just under the surface. If the pouch becomes infected, this artery can be damaged, and the resulting haemorrhage is extensive and difficult to control.

SAD (Small Airway Disease)

Small Airway Disease (SAD) or Chronic Obstructive Pulmonary Disease (COPD) is the next condition that our endoscope may meet as its exploration of the respiratory tract continues. As it travels down the trachea, it reveals the pools of thick, tacky mucus typical of this complaint. If the endoscope were thin enough to pass into the bronchioles, we would notice that the airways are clogged with excess mucus; the walls of the finer bronchioles are inflamed and thickened and the alveoli, the little air sacs at the end of the bronchioles, are over-inflated. We would also notice that the walls of the larger bronchioles are in spasm, causing a marked narrowing of the lumen (the

airspace inside the tube). The clogging effect of the mucus, the inflamed, thickened walls and the narrowing of the lumen of the bronchioles all drastically impede the free passage of air.

Researchers at Edinburgh Veterinary School used these facts to investigate a group of SAD horses. They found that there was a positive correlation between the development of the clinical, pathological and physical signs mentioned above and the horse's exposure to moulds in hay and bedding. Two moulds in particular were incriminated – *aspergillus fumigatus* and *micropolyspora faeni* – long names for the grey dust which billows out when badly made hay is shaken up.

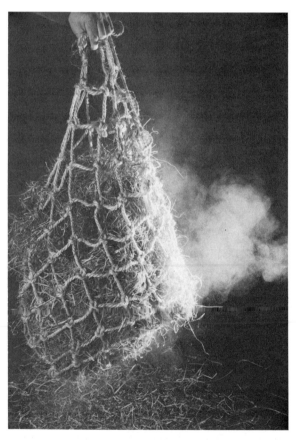

Fig 24 A cloud of dust shaken from medium quality hay. What chance have the horse's lungs?

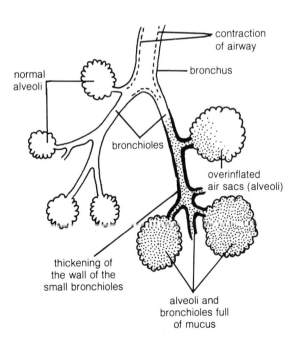

Fig 23 Changes in the lungs of a horse infected by SAD.

In a controlled environment, researchers showed that susceptible horses developed the disease within hours of exposure. More importantly, they discovered that SAD is reversible; remove the horse from the contaminated environment and the symptoms disappear. These horses became clinically normal in a short time.

We are reasonably certain that the fungal moulds which enter the lung with each breath can cause considerable reaction in sensitive horses. The greater the number of moulds present, and the longer the susceptible horse is exposed to these antigens, the more serious the reaction.

Instead of the horse standing quietly in the stable with respiratory movements hardly noticeable, he will be out of breath, wheezing badly and sometimes almost grunting with the effort of expelling the last bit of inhaled air. A long line, called the 'heave line', appears between the abdomen and chest wall, hence the old name for this condition, the 'heaves'. Even horses hardly affected by the condition show some signs of breathlessness. All have a chronic cough with harsh lung sounds, most have an increased respiratory rate and a double expiratory effort. Exercise tolerance is decreased and performance does not meet expectation.

Control of SAD This leads us on to the more practical aspects of the disease and how we control it. We know that exposure to moulds is the key factor. Remove the dust and SAD is eliminated, but how do we do this?

The best way of controlling SAD is to keep the horse out at all times and to feed him on a hay-free diet. Failing this, a dry, clean, airy stable is the first consideration. It is no use spending money on expensive, dust-free food and bedding unless the stable is well ventilated. This can be achieved by making sure that the stable is adequately insulated, thus keeping it warm and dry, and adequately ventilated, with inlet and outlet vents of the right size and correctly placed. The traditional stable, with its chimney trunk extractor and hopper inlets, satisfies these requirements adequately.

Probably the simplest stabling system is the lean-to shed, an open-fronted shed which is higher at the front than at the back, with the roof generally extending past the front of the stable to provide shade and shelter. Facing due south and protected from cold winds, with simple hopper inlets in the back wall, all stale air flows up and out at the front, to be replaced by clean air from the back and door areas. This simple system fulfils all the criteria for a warm and well-ventilated stable.

Having acquired a suitable stable, the next task is to prevent the living area from being contaminated by moulds and spores. To do this, a radical change in bedding and feeding habits may need to be undertaken. When a sensitised horse comes into contact with these antigens, the reaction is immediate. The greater the challenge, the worse the reaction so no moulds, no dust, and hopefully no SAD. Shredded paper, peat or coarse shavings used as a bedding material ensure that no antigens rise from the floor. It is important to make sure that the material, whatever it is, does not turn into a deep litter bed, as under suitable conditions the fungae can grow in this material as quickly as they do in straw.

A complete concentrate feed, or the use of ensiled, plastic-bagged hay or grass, will minimise antigens inhaled from the food. Of course, the whole campaign fails dismally if the normal horse next door spreads his stable dust into the poor SAD sufferer's air space. Hay and straw carried in front of the stable can also initiate symptoms, so keep the SAD horse isolated from his normal companions, or change the environment for them all.

Treatment of SAD Unfortunately we do not live in a perfect world, and occasionally the carefully managed SAD horse is allowed to come into contact with the dreaded moulds, generally when he is taken from his normal environment to a show or event. What can be done to protect him from this challenge or to treat the condition if it has already occurred?

Here we turn to recent advances made in the medical treatment of human asthma. Three groups of drugs are used. One group decreases the viscosity (thickness) of the mucus produced in the bronchioles, thus making it easier to expel the mucus and clear the airway. Another group acts on the constricted bronchioles and relaxes them, thus allowing a free passage of air into and out of the lungs. The third group acts on the cells involved in the reaction, desensitising them. Consequently the moulds do not cause any reaction and the lungs remain clear and functional. This last group has the added advantage of prolonged action, and two days' treatment protects the horse for up to ten days.

So far we have considered disorders of the respiratory system which affect the horse by reducing the amount of oxygen that reaches his lungs and therefore his tissues. The effects of those conditions are self-limiting – the horse gets less oxygen, so can do less work, but the only thing that suffers is performance. A different group of conditions which affect the horse's respiratory system are those diseases caused by infectious agents.

INFECTIOUS RESPIRATORY DISEASES

Bacterial Diseases

In the heyday of the working horse, bacterial diseases were much more common than they are now, as effective ways of controlling them had not been developed. Horses were kept in greater concentrations and epidemics would regularly sweep through whole populations.

Strangles Strangles is caused by bacteria called *Streptococcus equi* which affects young animals more than old, especially when they are grouped in large numbers. The disease is introduced to this susceptible population by an individual who carries the bacteria without showing any clinical signs of strangles. Under these conditions, the bacteria spreads very rapidly, either by direct contact between horses, or from contaminated food, buckets, etc. The bacteria can stay alive in infected premises for up to one year. All of a susceptible population can be infected, but the mortality rate is generally very low.

To prevent the spread of strangles, immediate isolation is necessary. This includes separate tack, feeding utensils, a separate groom to look after the sick animal and, of course, separate drainage and air space. However, the organism is so infectious that it may not be practical to attempt to control its spread under stud conditions.

The organism gains entry through the pharynx and rapidly infects the local lymph glands, especially those which lie between the lower jaw-bones. The horse develops a very sore throat and swallowing becomes difficult. At this stage, the temperature is generally very high, the horse looks ill, does not eat or drink and a thick discharge of mucus appears at the nostrils. The lymph glands between the jaw-bones – the submandibular glands – become hot and painful, swell up and eventually burst, releasing copious amounts of evil-smelling pus.

Once the glands have burst, the swelling rapidly diminishes, the pain and fever disappear and the horse starts to recover. The best form of treatment is, in fact, not to treat. *Strep. equi* is susceptible to most antibiotics and theoretically antibiotic therapy should cure the condition, but all too often, the use of antibiotics drives the infection to more inaccessible parts of the body where a form of strangles known as bastard strangles can develop. Abscesses form in the chest or in the abdomen, where they are almost impossible to treat. If antibiotics are to be used, the drug of choice is penicillin which should be given in large doses

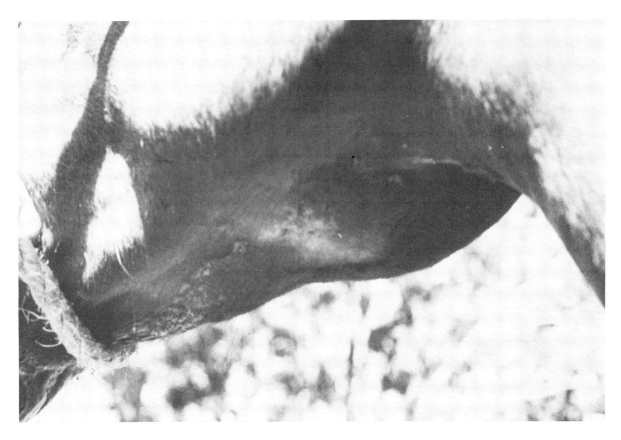

Fig 25   A typical strangles abscess on the underside of the lower jaw.

for at least seven days after the abscess has burst. A vaccine can be used to protect horses against the disease, but it is not without side-effects; it is available in the United States and Australia but not in Britain.

The most important part of the treatment is good nursing. The sick horse should be isolated in a warm, dry stable. In the early stages, the application of hot, damp towels to the swollen neck will ease the pain and encourage the maturation of the abscess. Once this has burst, which should take about four days, frequent bathing with hot water will assist drainage and encourage healing.

Glanders   Glanders is one of the few diseases of the horse which can cause a serious, often fatal disease in man. Fortunately, it has been eradicated in Britain, but with the rapid international movement of horses, it is as well to remember that it is still common in some other countries, including the United States.

Glanders is caused by bacteria called *Pseudomonas mallei*. This organism causes an acute pneumonia with a dry cough, a high temperature and a nasal discharge. In the horse, the condition can become chronic, with small nodules developing in the lungs and associated lymph glands. The horse has a foul-smelling nasal discharge and rapidly loses weight. A cutaneous (skin) form (farcy) also exists. Nodules develop in the skin, ulcerate quickly and discharge a grey-yellow pus. Due to the considerable risk to humans, treatment is not advisable.

49

Foal pneumonia Pneumonia can be defined as an infection of the lungs. Many agents can cause such an infection, most of them as a secondary development of a systemic disease. The pneumonia which occasionally follows strangles or influenza is a good example.

Bacteria called *Corynebacteria equi*, however, can cause a particularly nasty pneumonia in foals. The organism is found in soil and infection seems to be caused by the inhalation of contaminated dust. The infection is common in hot, dry environments, and is thought to be due to the large amounts of dust inhaled in these conditions. In the United States the disease is much more common than in Britain, where high rainfall, wet summers and lack of dust may be reasons why it is rare.

The infected foal gradually loses condition and a chronic cough develops. The whole progress of the disease is insidious. Frequently the foal has appeared quite well until just before death. The mortality rate is high, 60-70 per cent and, to be successful, treatment must be started in the early stages of the condition.

Viral Diseases

For the last decade, the viruses which infect the respiratory tract have assumed greater significance as the causal agents of disease. The reason may be our greater understanding of the infecting agent, the virus, and its effect on the host, the horse. Another factor, of increasing importance, may be the much greater movement of horses from population to population. Horse-boxes can take a symptomless carrier from one yard suffering from the ubiquitous 'virus' to another yard as yet free from infection in a matter of a few hours. If this yard, or show, or local meet has a high proportion of horses with a low immunity to that virus, the next outbreak of the disease has already started.

Equine influenza Equine influenza is caused by two strains of the type-A influenza virus

They are named after the cities where they were first isolated. Hence we have type-A/equi/Prague 56, first discovered in Czechoslovakia during 1956 and type-A/equi/Miami 63, isolated in 1963 from ill horses in Miami, Florida. These two strains cause similar symptoms in the horse, but are immunologically distinct. A horse who has recovered from the Prague strain has an immunity to this strain but not to the Miami strain. In the last few years new strains have been discovered, an example of which is the strain type-A/equi/Newmarket 79, which caused outbreaks of flu in vaccinated horses during 1979–80. New strains are incorporated in the flu vaccines in an attempt to extend the range of immunity that they give.

Equine influenza is an acute respiratory disease. The virus gains entry through the nose and attacks the lining of the trachea and bronchioles causing damage and eventual death of large areas of the mucosa (mucous membranes). The incubation period is short, three to four days. Poor ventilation which increases the concentration of viral particles, together with the above characteristics, ensure the explosive spread of the disease.

In the older horse the main symptoms are a high temperature, a clear nasal discharge and a cough. In the absence of secondary infection with bacteria, the mucosa can regenerate in three weeks. However, the muscle of the heart can also be damaged, so complete rest for up to six weeks is essential. Young animals can be so badly affected that the primary viral infection can cause death, but more usually a secondary pneumonia caused by a *streptococcus* species is the cause of death. The incidence of SAD in horses that have had flu is also much higher. Frequently, horses become allergic to moulds after a flu attack.

There is no doubt that the introduction of flu vaccines, and especially the compulsory vaccination of all racehorses, and later of all competing horses, has reduced the incidence of flu to minimal levels. However, the ability of the virus to throw up new strains which may not be covered by present vaccines means that we cannot afford to be complacent.

In Great Britain, the official influenza vaccination requirements for any horse engaged in racing are that a primary vaccination should be followed by a second vaccination, not less than 21 days and not more than 92 days after the primary. Horses born after 1 January 1980 must receive a further booster vaccination not less than 150 days and not more than 215 days after the second vaccination. Annual boosters must be given. Annual boosters given before 16 March 1981 must not exceed 14 months, and after this date must not exceed 12 months.

Although FEI (Federation Equestre International) rules do not require that horses born after 1980 should have the extra booster, it is as well to remember that any horse entering racecourse premises must be vaccinated according to Jockey Club rules. In fact, the increasing vaccination requirements of all major equestrian events mean that competitors should ensure that all vaccination details are recorded on one of the new identification/vaccination cards. The British Horse Society Riding Club newsletter *A guide to current equine influenza vaccine rules* is an excellent summary of the complicated requirements for competition.

In spite of the adverse publicity attached to this compulsory scheme, mostly due to the extra cost involved and the idea that vaccination can adversely affect performance, there is no doubt that it is removing influenza as an economically important disease in horses.

Equine rhinovirus The rhinovirus of the horse can be compared with the virus which causes the common cold in humans. It causes a transient disease more common in young horses who have been moved into a close association with older horses. It is characterised by a copious nasal discharge and a temperature rise, both of which generally disappear in a few days.

Equine rhinopneumonitis The virus which causes rhinopneumonitis belongs to the Herpes group. Two subtypes known as EHV-I type 1 and EHV-I type 2 both cause respiratory symptoms. The EHV-I type 1 virus can also cause abortions and paralysis.

Before 1979 it was thought that the common type in Great Britain was the type 2 virus which caused a transient disease in young horses, especially when they were collected into large groups after weaning. Once infected, the horse develops a high temperature with a slight, clear nasal discharge. The glands

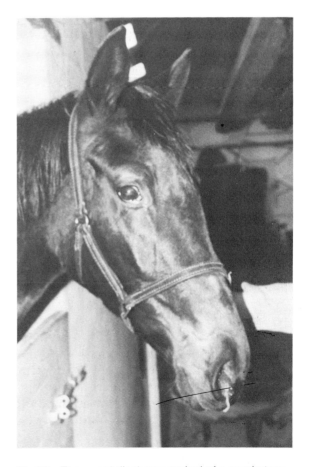

Fig 26 The nasal discharge typical of a respiratory infection in a young animal.

of the head and neck sometimes become enlarged and the clear discharge can become mucopurulent, thick, grey–yellow and smelly, as secondary infection takes place. More seriously, performance can be badly affected and horses can take up to three months to return to their previous level of fitness.

Since then, cases of the more dangerous type 1 infection have occurred. During 1979, a group of mares, foals and three stallions became infected after one mare in the group aborted. The first sign noticed was a mild fever lasting about three days, followed by a period of inappetance (lack of appetite) and within seven days, 50 per cent of the population had developed varying degrees of ataxia (paralysis of the hind quarters). Nine mares had to be put down. Since this incident, many other cases of type 1 abortion have been reported and it appears that the type 1 virus may be as common as the type 2, causing a similar type of respiratory infection in young horses and abortion and paralysis in older horses.

As with all virus diseases, there is no cure for rhinopneumonitis. The only way of controlling the disease is to stop it spreading by prompt isolation of all aborting mares and by thorough cleaning and disinfection of the contaminated area. Any animals in contact with the infection should also be isolated and all movement to and from the infected premises should be halted until the outbreak is over.

Two vaccines are now available in Britain. A live vaccine which is licenced for use against respiratory infection only, and a dead vaccine which can be used to protect breeding mares and animals in contact with the infection against abortions. Due to the low level of immunity produced by the dead vaccine, it has to be given at least three times during pregnancy to be effective. Both vaccines use the type 1 strain and therefore give little immunity against disease caused by the type 2 virus. Vaccines are also available in the United States.

Equine viral arteritis Luckily this is another viral disease which has not reared its ugly head in Britain, although it causes sporadic outbreaks in the United States. The virus attacks the muscle layer of small arteries, especially those in the lungs, and in the pregnant uterus. The first signs are a temperature rise, a nasal discharge and usually a severe conjunctivitis. The legs and areas under the abdomen can become swollen. Sometimes the damage to the arteries causes diarrhoea and abortion is a common complication. An experimental vaccine has been tested in the United States but is not commercially available. There is no cure for the disease, but good nursing and supportive treatment ensure that the mortality rate remains low.

Parasitic Disease

Parascaris equorum The larvae of the large white worm *Parascaris equorum* pass through the lungs during their migration through the body of the young horse, before growing into adult worms in the small intestine. If the infestation is a heavy one, large numbers of larvae can damage the lining of the bronchial tubes, causing a nasty cough and a smelly nasal discharge. This occurs in foals between four and six months in age and although the disease is rarely serious it can predispose the foal to infection with more dangerous agents.

Lungworm Lungworm (*Dictyocaulus arnfieldi*) breed in the lungs of the donkey. In this species they live without causing much disease and lay large numbers of eggs which contaminate the pasture. Horses grazing this pasture eat the eggs which hatch out in the intestine. They migrate to the lungs where, with few exceptions, they remain as infertile worms unable to complete their life cycle, but causing a chronic, non-productive cough.

Lungworm infection should be suspected in any horse who has a chronic cough at rest and at exercise, and who grazes in company with donkeys or in a field in which donkeys have grazed. As the eggs of *dictyocaulus* are very resistant to climatic changes, the period over which the pasture is infective can last for years after the donkeys have left.

Treatment is simple. All donkeys should be regularly wormed with a wormer which is effective against lungworm; similarly, any horse out at pasture who has a chronic cough should also receive a good worming. Effective wormers are Equalan, Equitac or Systamex and large doses of Panacur.

6 Circulatory System

The circulatory system can be thought of as the transport system of the body. Within a network of blood vessels and pumped by the heart, the blood moves carbohydrates and proteins from the digestive tract to the organs that need them. It transports the oxygen that the body uses to burn food, thus producing the energy that the body requires, and it also takes the waste products produced from this reaction to the lungs, kidneys and gut, where they are excreted. As well as transporting these materials around the body, the circulatory system contains in the blood a whole series of specialised cells responsible for the body's defence.

STRUCTURE OF THE CIRCULATORY SYSTEM

The centre of the circulatory system is the heart. In the horse this is a large, powerful muscular organ that lies in the chest surrounded by a tough fibrous sac called the pericardium. The blood vessels that carry the blood to all parts of the body start out from the heart as high-pressure, elastic-sided tubes called arteries. These spread in a branching network through the tissues, becoming narrower as they go, until they become microscopic tubules called capillaries.

It is through the thin walls of the capillaries that the blood takes up and then releases its store of nutrients and oxygen and absorbs the waste products of energy production. Once through the capillary network the blood is returned to the heart by a system of low-pressure, thin-walled vessels called veins.

The heart consists of four chambers, the left and right atria (upper chambers) and the left and right ventricles (lower chambers). Blood from the right side of the heart is pumped from the right ventricle through the lungs, where oxygen is taken up and carbon dioxide excreted, and returned via the pulmonary veins to the left side. The richly oxygenated blood, now bright red in colour, passes from the left atrium into the left ventricle and is pumped at high pressure through the arteries, then the narrower arterioles and finally through the capillary network where the oxygen is extracted by those tissues that need it. Once through the capillary network the blood is returned to the heart via the veins. They empty into the right atrium and the darker deoxygenated blood passes from the atrium into the right ventricle where, once more, it is pumped through the lungs.

A system of blood vessels called the portal veins short circuits this cycle. They take blood, enriched with nutrients, from the gut to the liver. Here the nutrients are broken down to carbohydrates, fat and amino acids and rejoin the general circulation, to be used by the tissues as they are required.

BLOOD

Which of the blood's constituents allow it to perform so many functions?

We all think of blood as a sticky, thick red substance that clots when it is released from the body, but in reality it is far more complex. It consists of a straw-coloured fluid called plasma, in which are suspended many microscopic cells. The plasma, together with the intra and extracellular fluid in the tissue, forms the water reservoir of the horse. The amino acids and carbohydrates that the body tissues need are carried by the plasma, in solution.

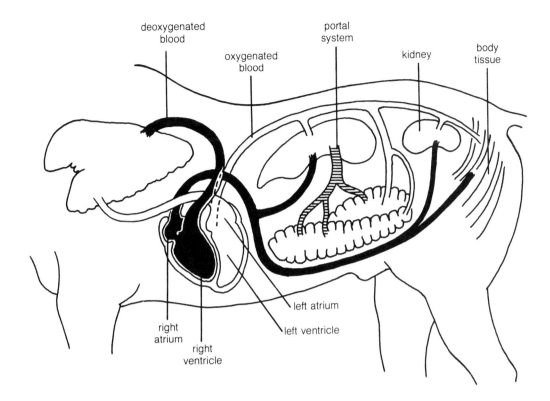

Fig 27 The circulatory system.

The fat, a very useful fuel, is transported as a fine suspension of globules.

The red colour of the blood is due to large quantities of specialised cells called red blood cells or erythrocytes. Each erythrocyte contains an organic iron compound and a protein which together make a pigment called haemoglobin. Where the oxygen levels are high, such as in the lungs, haemoglobin combines with oxygen to form a bright red compound called oxyhaemoglobin. Then, where oxygen levels are low, such as in working tissues, the oxyhaemoglobin releases its oxygen. The reverse happens to the waste product carbon dioxide. This is taken up by the haemoglobin where the concentration is high, as in working tissues, and is released in the lungs where the concentration is low. This process takes place rapidly, which is just as well as each red blood cell takes only a second to traverse the capillary network, very little time in which to release the amount of oxygen that hard-working tissues need.

Another group of cells found in the blood is called the white blood cells. There are five types of white cells; the most common two, lymphocytes and neutrophils account for 70 per cent to 95 per cent of the total, eosinophils, monocytes and basophils make up the rest. White blood cells are the front line troops in the defence mechanisms of the horse.

The most common white cell, the neutrophil, attacks bacteria. In response to a bacterial challenge, the number of neutrophils increases markedly. Each neutrophil attempts to fold itself around a bacterium, an action called phagocytosis. Unfortunately this action often kills the neutrophil as well as the bacterium. The collection of dead cells and bacteria, together with plasma and damaged tissue make up what

55

we know as pus.

Lymphocytes are more concerned with producing antibodies, those proteins which have the job of neutralising viruses and bacteria.

The exact functions of the less common white blood cells are not clear. Eosinophils are found in association with an allergic reaction and also rise in numbers during a parasitic attack. Monocytes are found in more chronic infections and concentrate on mopping up dead bacteria and cell debris.

A third type of cell particle, called platelets, also circulates in the blood system. These cells are an essential link in the complex process of blood clotting. The platelets have a knack of seeking out small breaks in the walls of the capillary vessels and, by settling in the gap, soon plug the defect.

DISEASES OF THE CIRCULATORY SYSTEM

The diseases that affect the circulatory system can be divided into those which cause a condition of the blood called anaemia, and those disorders of the heart and vessels which influence the flow of blood around the body.

Anaemia

How often have you seen some 'expert' look at a horse and say 'he's pale in the eye, he must be anaemic'? Unfortunately anaemia is not a disease in its own right but a symptom. It demands a thorough examination of the horse and a detailed laboratory examination of his blood before the underlying cause of the anaemia can be determined.

Anaemia can be defined as a shortage of haemoglobin in the blood. This can be as a result of a reduction in the number of circulating red blood cells, or by a reduction in the haemoglobin concentration in those cells, or a combination of both. It only occurs as part of some other condition.

One form of anaemia arises after an acute haemorrhage. If the horse has lost a lot of blood due to a cut, or a major operation, then the total number of blood cells in the body falls rapidly. The haemoglobin concentration in each cell is normal but the number of cells in each millilitre of blood is low. In these cases the bone marrow, where most erythrocytes are produced, is stimulated to produce more cells and the red blood cells can be back to normal numbers in approximately three weeks.

A chronic blood loss, however, can outstrip the horse's ability to produce new blood cells or to fill the cells with the normal amount of haemoglobin. This type of anaemia is common in horses with a heavy worm burden. The redworm of the horse is a blood sucker, and in the young or old horse can rapidly produce a severe anaemia by exhausting the bone marrow's ability to produce enough new red blood cells. In more severe cases, the body's reserves of iron are exhausted. Iron is an essential part of haemoglobin, so no iron, no haemoglobin. The result is a severe, iron deficient anaemia which takes a long time to correct. Parasites such as lice and ticks also suck blood and when they are present in large numbers are capable of causing this type of anaemia.

Haemolytic disease of the foal causes another type of anaemia. This acute anaemia is caused by antibodies present in the mother's milk which destroy the foal's own red blood cells.

Luckily in Great Britain there are no infectious diseases which specifically affect the blood system. However, one such disease, equine infectious anaemia, is common in other parts of the world. The disease is caused by a virus which attacks the liver and causes a dramatic fall in red blood cell numbers and in the haemoglobin level of the blood. The disease is incurable and those horses that survive the acute attack can become symptomless carriers. Luckily a reliable test called the 'Coggins test' can detect these carriers, and the requirement that international travellers must be negative to this test should prevent the spread of the disease.

If we believed the literature of some makers of iron tonics and vitamin preparations, we would suppose that the horse can quite easily develop an anaemia due to a vitamin or iron deficiency. In fact, the levels of iron and vitamins in the normal feed of a horse are quite adequate and anaemia due to a lack of these substances is rare. A temporary anaemia can occasionally occur in the horse who is undergoing a strenuous training programme. The extra blood cells needed to cope with the extra work can use up available stores of iron and vitamin B12 and these substances may then have to be added to the diet.

The lack of one other vitamin in the diet can cause anaemia. Folic acid plays an essential part in the production of both red and white blood cells. Folic acid is found in plenty in fresh grass but disappears as grass is made into hay. Horses who spend a long time in stables, fed on a diet of hard food and hay can become deficient. The anaemia that develops can be cured by the addition of folic acid to the diet or can be prevented by feeding alfalfa or silage, both rich sources of this vitamin.

Anaemia, then, is a condition typified by a low concentration of haemoglobin in the blood. This means that the blood cannot carry its normal amount of oxygen and the tissues become starved of oxygen. Oxygen is necessary to produce energy, so the picture that we see in an anaemic horse is that of a weak, lethargic animal who performs badly. In an anaemic state the heart muscle, which needs lots of oxygen, does not work efficiently, it tires easily, and a heart murmur develops. The appetite is depressed and the hair becomes dull and lifeless but it is not until the anaemia becomes severe that the mucous membranes appear pale.

Heart Disease

The heart is a pump and in a sequence of contractions it squeezes the blood from one chamber to another and on into the arteries. To prevent the blood from flowing backwards, the heart is equipped with valves between the atria and ventricles and at the entrance to the two main arteries leaving the heart. It is the noise of these valves opening and shutting – the familiar 'luub dup', 'luub dup' – that we hear when we listen to the heart. Occasionally, due to disease or congenital defect, the valves do not close properly. When this happens the smooth flow of the blood is interrupted and turbulence occurs. We hear this as a roaring sound between the normal heart sounds and by pinpointing its position relative to the heart sounds, we can tell which valve is faulty.

The rhythm of the heart is controlled by a group of specialised nodes, the pacemakers, which initiate and then control the waves of stimulation which spread across the heart, making first the atria contract and then the ventricles.

When a horse is at rest, with the heart just ticking over, it is quite common to find that the occasional beat is missed. The pacemaker has forgotten to send out its signal. As soon as the horse starts to exercise or becomes excited, the pacemaker concentrates on its task and the rhythm becomes normal. This is quite a common condition and does not seem to affect performance in any way.

A more worrying condition occurs when the pacemaker sends out a constant stream of impulses to the atria which respond by fibrillating (making lots of partial contractions). This condition, known as atrial fibrillation, has a profound effect upon performance. The atria fail to contract as a whole and therefore do not pump sufficient blood into the ventricles. They, in their turn, have a fast erratic beat and a low output of blood. Very often further pathological change is found in the valves or heart muscle. The drug quinidine sulphate, which is given by mouth, will sometimes arrest the arrhythmia and return the heart to normal function.

We are all used to a veterinary surgeon examining a horse's heart with a stethoscope. By listening to the heart sounds, especially the relationship between the sound and its position, he can identify many heart lesions present. However, to predict the likely significance is much more difficult.

The horse with the occasional dropped beat which becomes regular with exercise is no problem, and he is quite sound. Nor is the horse with a gross heart lesion and associated changes in the body a problem, as he is obviously ill. It is the large number of other cases with a heart lesion but no other obvious change that are difficult. We have all heard of the faithful hunter who was condemned by the vet as having a 'dicky heart', who still hunts twice a week and has done so for many years. Even the use of an electrocardiogram and a phonocardiogram, the former recording the electrical impulses which pass through the heart muscle and the latter the noise of the heart beat, only assist us in making a more accurate diagnosis. A large percentage of horses still remain where we have to say: 'he has a heart lesion but it is questionable how significant it is.' In view of the serious consequences for the rider if a horse should collapse, it is not surprising that we err on the side of caution.

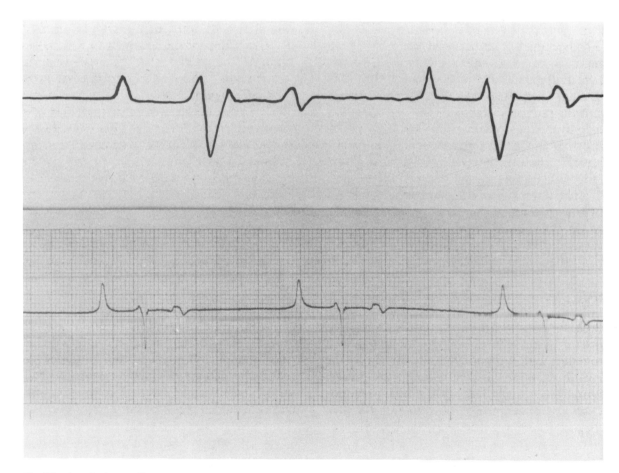

Fig 28   An electrocardiogram trace.

DISEASE OF THE BLOOD VESSELS

Due to the horse's healthy diet – plenty of roughage and no saturated fatty acids – disease of the arteries such as that which occurs in humans, is rare in the horse. The only condition of importance is that caused by the migrating redworm larvae. They can cause a weak area in the wall of the artery, an aneurism, which then balloons rather like a badly patched inner tube and, like an inner tube, it can blow out with dire consequences. The massive haemorrhage which results causes an acute collapse, rapid unconsciousness and death.

THE LYMPHATIC SYSTEM

The lymphatic system consists of a branching network of thin-walled vessels which originate in the tissues and join together, eventually to empty into the main vein, the vena cava. At various points on this network lie collections of lymphocytes and connective tissue, which together make up structures called lymph nodes. The content of this system is a colourless fluid called lymph which, helped by a system of valves which prevent it from flowing backwards, moves slowly from the tissues along the lymph channels and through the lymph nodes to the main lymphatic vessel, and from there into the vena cava.

Functions

The function of the lymphatic system is primarily protective. Any foreign particles, together with lymphocytes, are carried by the lymph from the infected tissue to the nearest lymph node. Here, large cells similar to monocytes engulf the foreign particles and pass on a message to the lymphocytes warning them of the nature of the threat. The lymphocytes then manufacture an antibody which will neutralise other particles of a similar nature.

The lymphatic system, like the vascular system, also has a transport function. The lymph vessels from the intestines transport fat absorbed from the intestinal villi and take it to the vena cava where it joins the venous system.

Diseases of the Lymphatic System

Filling of the legs This condition is so common that it is more a nuisance than a disease. It occurs as a puffy swelling of the lower legs which develops during the period when the horse is resting, and it disappears as soon as exercise starts. The condition is more common in the fit, well-fed horse and local bruising will increase the amount of fluid present. Lymph is moved from the extremities of the horse into the centre by a combination of pressure and the massaging effect of adjacent muscles. The absence of muscle, and the length of leg in the horse, mean that lymph finds it very difficult to move up the limb and, during rest, it stagnates and collects under the skin.

Lymphangitis This is a more serious sequel to filling of the legs. It is common in the hind legs and occurs when a cut becomes infected. The infection rapidly spreads up the lymphatic vessels causing a hot, painful swelling which can involve the whole leg. Lymph glands and vessels are particularly swollen and serous fluid oozes from the skin. The horse is obviously ill; he has a high temperature and is generally off his food. Prompt treatment with high doses of antibiotics, to control the infection, and phenylbutazone and diuretics, to reduce the inflammation and swelling, is necessary. Inadequately treated cases become chronic, leaving a thickened, scarred leg.

7 Reproductive System

FEMALE REPRODUCTIVE ORGANS

The female reproductive tract consists of two ovaries, the uterus, the cervix and the vagina and vulva.

The ovaries are organs which vary in size but are generally about 8cm long and 4cm broad. The main function of the ovaries is to develop specialised cells within their substance into female germ cells called the ova. When one of these cells is fully developed it is expelled from the ovary, a process known as ovulation. The ovary also produces important chemicals – hormones – which help to govern the process.

The whole period from the development of the egg, its subsequent shedding and the development of the next egg is called the oestrous cycle. The ovaries are connected to the rest of the reproductive tract by two tubes called the fallopian tubes. One end of the tube, that closest to the ovary, is funnel shaped and when the egg is released from the ovary the funnel guides the egg into the lumen of the fallopian tube where it starts its journey down the reproductive tract. The uterus comprises two horns into which the fallopian tubes open. The horns join together to form the body of the uterus. It is in this organ that fertilisation takes place and where the fertilised egg or embryo starts to develop into a foal.

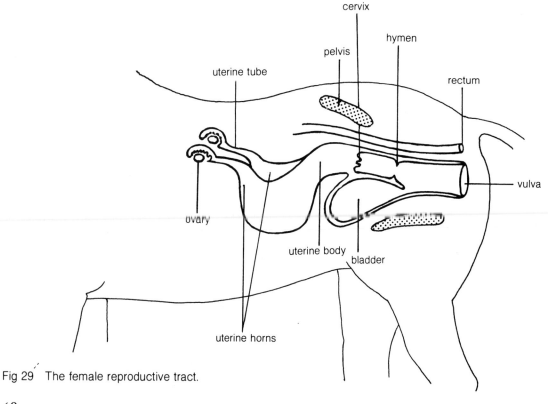

Fig 29 The female reproductive tract.

The uterus is connected to the outside by a tough-walled tube called the vagina. Between the two, protecting the uterus from outside contamination, is the cervix. The muscular walls of the cervix are greatly influenced by changing hormone levels during the oestrous cycle and its appearance is a great help in deciding the stage of the oestrous cycle. The whole tract, from ovaries to cervix is suspended from the backbone by a strong sheet of tissue called the broad ligament of the uterus.

MALE REPRODUCTIVE ORGANS

The reproductive tract of the male consists of two glands called the testicles. They are responsible for producing the spermatozoa – the male germ cell – and like the ovaries, they also produce hormones. In this case, the male hormone testosterone is predominant. Testosterone is responsible for the development of male characteristics – the heavy crest of the stallion – and it also controls the correct development of the secondary sex glands.

The spermatozoa develop in a system of tubules called seminiferous tubules which are in the testicle. The spermatozoa mature as they pass down the tubules and eventually enter a structure sitting on top of the testicle. This structure is called the epididymis and within its system of tubules the sperm undergo further development before they pass into the *vas deferens*. This is one of a pair of ducts carrying sperm from the testicle or epididymis to the outside, through the tube called the urethra in the penis. These tubes, one from each epididymis, pass into the body through the left and right inguinal rings and connect the testicle to the urethra. It is through the urethra that urine is passed from the bladder to the exterior and it is into this tube that secretions from the secondary sex glands – the seminal vesicles and the prostate – join with the sperm to form the ejaculate.

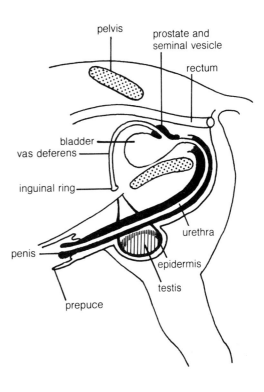

Fig 30   Male reproductive organs.

In order that the ejaculate reaches the uterus and the sperm fertilises the ova, the penis of the stallion has to become erect. This is achieved when the large spaces in the body of the penis, the corpus cavernosum, become engorged with blood. The penis rapidly enlarges and can now enter the vagina of the mare where ejaculation takes place.

ENVIRONMENT AND REPRODUCTION

Reproductive behaviour of both the mare and stallion is environmentally sensitive; that is, environmental factors, for example temperature, light and food supply, play an important role in the development of normal reproductive activity in both the male and female.

By nature the mare is seasonally polyoestrous – she has oestrous cycles during one period of the year. In the depths of winter she shows no oestrous behaviour and rectal palpation will show that the ovaries are small and hard. This condition is known as anoestrous. As the season advances into spring, the days get longer, the temperature increases and the food supply gets better. These early environmental changes have an effect on the hormone levels and reproductive organs of the mare and a transitional period, when the organs develop into full patency, takes place. The three conditions, food, temperature and increasing light – the environmental threshold – are at their most potent some time in May or June and it is then that the mare has developed a normal oestrous cycle and is at her most fertile.

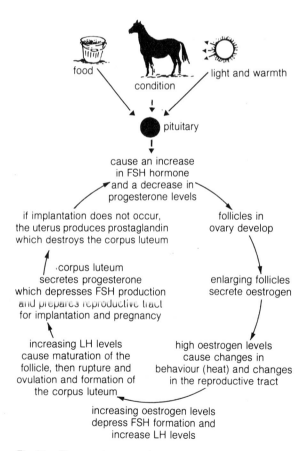

Fig 31   The oestrous cycle.

It is as well to remember that this cycle is arranged not for the mare's or for man's benefit, but to ensure that the foal is born at the best time for its own survival. As summer changes into autumn the mare sinks into a reverse transitional period, which finally leads to winter anoestrus. This period is of little importance to us, as by that time we hope the mare is safely in foal.

The stallion is also affected by the environmental threshold, but not to the same extent as the mare. Although he is fertile all the year around, it has been shown that during the winter months the sperm count declines and his libido is less.

THE OESTROUS CYCLE

The oestrous cycle of the mare is 20 to 22 days long. It is separated into oestrus which lasts 4 to 6 days, and dioestrus (the period between each oestrus) which lasts 16 days. The average mare shows that she is in oestrus by her behaviour. She passes frequent small amounts of urine, she is attracted to a stallion or gelding and shows this attraction by crouching. She raises her tail and contracts and expands the vulva and exerts the clitoris at the same time, an action called 'winking'. Her character changes; the placid mare often becomes irritable when in heat, although the reverse can happen and the difficult mare may become quiet.

How do these changes occur? A whole range of hormones – chemicals secreted by glands in the body – act and react with each other and with the reproductive organs in the body to produce the changes which happen during the oestrous cycle.

Under the influence of increasing light, heat and a rising plane of nutrition – the environmental threshold – a part of the brain called the hypothalamus secretes a group of hormones. This acts on a small gland tucked under the brain, called the pituitary gland and persuades

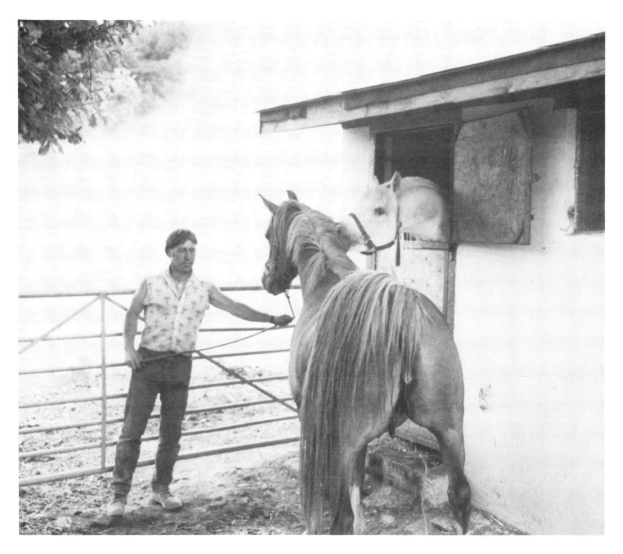

Fig 32 A mare in full oestrus, tail elevated and 'winking'.

it to secrete increasing amounts of a hormone called follicle stimulating hormone (FSH). FSH, in its turn, acts on the ovaries and stimulates the growth of underdeveloped follicles. These small, fluid-filled sacs each contain an egg or ovum and as they develop they secrete another hormone called oestrogen. It is this hormone which is responsible for the physical signs of heat, which are necessary before the mare will accept the stallion, and also for the changes which occur in the repro-

ductive tract. The cervix, the gate between the vagina and uterus, becomes relaxed and vascular and the walls of the vagina secrete a lubricant mucus. These changes help to ensure the safe passage of the stallion's sperm as it moves up the uterus to meet the descending egg.

The pituitary gland is constantly checking on the level of oestrogen in the blood and once a certain concentration has been reached it acts again. A further hormone, luteinising hormone (LH) is secreted. This firstly reduces the production of FSH and then, acting on the ovary, accelerates the development of one follicle, causing its eventual rupture and release of the ovum – a process called ovulation. Ovulation occurs about 24 hours before the end of oestrus.

How and why only one follicle is chosen we do not know. Sometimes, of course, two follicles mature and release two ova, which then develop into twins. The high incidence of twinning in the Thoroughbred and hence the high level of abortion is one reason for the relatively large number of empty Thoroughbred mares in the autumn.

Once ovulation has occurred the level of oestrogen produced by the follicle falls rapidly, the mare goes out of season and her reaction to the stallion changes. Any advances made by him now lead to the more usual behaviour of an out of season mare – biting, kicking and squealing.

The empty follicle develops into a specialised gland called the corpus luteum which secretes yet another hormone named progesterone. The function of progesterone is directed mainly at the uterus. It prepares this organ for the implantation of the fertilised ovum and ensures that the lining of the uterus is ready to maintain early pregnancy. It also reduces the amount of FSH secreted from the pituitary gland, thus slowing down the development of new follicles.

The uterus now takes a hand in the management of the cycle. If fertilisation has not taken place and implantation has not occurred, the uterus produces a hormone called prostaglandin. This destroys the corpus luteum in the ovary and the level of progesterone produced by this gland falls rapidly. The orchestrator of the cycle – the pituitary gland – senses this drop and in reply increases the amount of FSH hormone which acts on the ovary, stimulating the growth of the next crop of follicles. In this way the cycle repeats itself.

MANAGEMENT

The Normal Mare

Within the normal breeding season, between May and August, very few problems should occur. The signs of heat are very evident, the stallion should be virile and the mare fertile, and the only problem is knowing when ovulation has occurred. The average date quoted in various reference books is given as the last or second last day of oestrus; oestrus lasts approximately 4 days in mid season and longer at the beginning and end of the season. Once ovulation has occurred, the ovum has a life of 36 hours and the sperm must be in the female reproductive tract for 8 hours before it is able to fertilise the egg. Timing is therefore of the utmost importance. How do we judge this time?

The individuals concerned know best. Their behaviour towards one another can be used to judge when the mare is most fertile. The process is known as teasing; the mare is introduced to the stallion, generally over a partition, and their reactions to each other are noted. If the mare is ready to be mated the stallion makes it clear by showing a peculiar facial grimace known as 'flehmen' in which the top lip is curled back to reveal the incisor teeth, and although the mare may exhibit token resistance, she soon becomes acquiescent. Young maiden mares need special care – it is all too easy to frighten them so much that mating becomes a permanently traumatic experience. Mares with young foals often override their sexual response because of their intense maternal instinct. This can lead to a long, drawn out teasing before her mating instincts become stronger than her maternal anxiety and normal heat behaviour occurs.

As a general rule a mare should be served 2 days after the onset of heat and again 2 days later, in this way we can be sure that a viable ova meets a healthy sperm and fertilisation will take place.

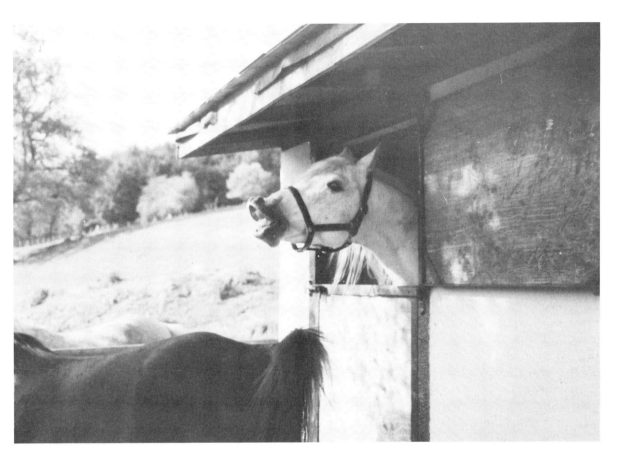

Fig 33   Typical 'flehmen' shown by a stallion. The mare's cocked tail indicates her readiness.

The Abnormal Mare

The problem of timing becomes more difficult when attempts are made to breed early in the year. The official birth date for Thoroughbred foals is January, which means that it is advantageous to start breeding mares in February – the earlier the foal is born after January, the more physically developed he will be when he eventually has to perform, whether on the racetrack or in the show ring. Unfortunately a high proportion of mares are still in the transition period and their oestrus cycle is irregular, ovulation is often absent and even if the mare is covered successfully, fertilisation may not occur.

As has already been mentioned, environmental influences have a great effect on the cycle and in the early spring the ovaries start to wake up. The delicate balance that exists between the emergence of normal oestrus behaviour and the environmental threshold can explain the erratic behaviour of the barren or maiden mare at this time. This behaviour can vary from an inactive mare with some follicle development in the ovaries, to ovarian activity and ovulation with no signs of heat, to those puzzling mares who show some ovarian activity and irregular periods of heat, sometimes only for a day. The varying changes which occur during the transition period can be best explained by imagining the mare to be hovering just under the environmental threshold. Every now and again, the weather or her improving condition allows her to rise above this level and heat develops for a short time before disappearing as she sinks below the threshold again. Other mares remain above the threshold level but the follicle takes a long time to develop because the environment is still not suitable. These mares are commonly in heat for the whole period, up to six weeks.

Eventually, as the season progresses, the all-important environmental changes are strong enough to iron out all these irregularities and a normal cycle occurs. The cycle is then repeated throughout the season until in the autumn the decreasing light, colder weather and reduced food supply bring in the last period, the transition into anoestrus.

The reverse happens to the hunter mare or the chaser being brought up to full fitness in the autumn. In these cases, just as the mare would normally be moving towards anoestrus, she is rapidly improving in condition and being fed larger quantities of food. These stimuli can be strong enough to overwhelm the effect of the reduction in daylight and encourage the development of a normal oestrous cycle.

What happens when a fit and well-fed mare is retired to stud? Most mares are let down, the environmental factors then take charge, the environmental threshold is rapidly lowered and just when normal oestrous cycles are wanted, they vanish. How are we going to get a mare in foal during this confusing time? The first priority is to examine the patient internally to find out what is happening to her oestrus cycle. Once this is known then treatment can be started.

Anoestrus Mares

If she is in true anoestrus, that is, she shows no ovarian activity, there is little that can be done. Using artificial light to increase the hours of daylight to at least 16 hours a day, together with extra food and warmth will sometimes allow her to rise above the environmental threshold and ensure the start of some ovarian activity. The injection of the hormone that stimulates the production of FSH and LH can produce some ovarian activity but much more work has yet to be done before truly anoestrus mares can be persuaded to develop normal cycles.

Mares in the Transitional Period

In mares where there is some ovarian activity, an orally active synthetic progesterone, given as a food supplement called Regumate, can be used to 'regulate' the cycle and ensure a normal heat and ovulation. The synthetic progesterone acts on the pituitary gland preventing the release of LH. When the treatment ends, the regulatory effect of Regumate ends and a bounce-back effect allows a high level of LH to be released. This ensures the development of a good follicle, ovulation and a normal heat.

Mares with a foal at foot, as well as being shy when teased, can go for a long time with no apparent heat periods. With the present high cost of keeping a mare at stud it is essential to bring these mares on and cover them as soon as possible.

Lactation Anoestrus

This condition is caused by high levels of the hormone prolactin which stimulates the let-down of milk. In some mares these levels are high enough to create anoestrus. Less affected mares suffer from a persistent corpus luteum which, by maintaining a high level of progesterone, prevents heat developing. An injection of prostaglandin will destroy the corpus luteum allowing a normal heat to develop. In extreme cases the ovaries show very little activity and the best treatment is to start a course of Regumate and give an injection of prostaglandin on the last day of treatment.

INFERTILITY DUE TO ACUTE INFECTION

Infection of the uterus (endometritis) can occur as a result of damage at foaling, it is often a sequel to a retained placenta and of course can be a sexually transmitted disease such as Contagious equine metritis (CEM).

Contagious Equine Metritis

This disease is caused by bacteria called *Haemophilus equigenitalia* and was first recognised in Ireland during the 1976 season. It is a sexually transmitted disease carried by symptomless mares or stallions. The typical disease is characterised by a profuse vaginal discharge occurring 24-48 hours after service. This becomes less over the next 10 days but inflammation of the cervix remains and can cause infertility. Antibiotic treatment, both parenteral and local, is needed to cure the condition (parenteral treatment is the administration of a substance other than via the digestive system, for example by injection).

Other bacteria can cause acute infection of the vagina and uterus and any discharge from the vagina, either after foaling or service, should be checked immediately. Early treatment means early cure and a quick return to normal fertility. Because of the severe economic effect of the disease, a system of sampling mares and stallions before breeding has been developed. Routine swabs are taken of the cervix, the most effective time being when the mare is in heat. The clitoral fossa, at the entrance to the vagina, is a favourite lurking place of the CEM organism and should be swabbed. Stallions are checked by examining washings taken from the prepuce (foreskin of the penis). The routine checking of mares and stallions in this way has reduced the incidence of the disease markedly.

Coital Exanthema (Horse Pox)

Coital exanthema is an acute disease, also sexually transmitted, caused by a member of the herpes virus family. Numerous vesicles (small blisters) develop on the external genitalia, the prepuce and penis of the stallion and the vulval lips of the mare. Secondary infection leads to acute inflammation and a vaginal discharge. The disease does not appear to cause infertility and the individual case recovers in 3 to 4 weeks.

INFERTILITY DUE TO CHRONIC INFECTION

The chronic disease is less obvious and failure to come into heat due to the persistence of a corpus luteum is the most common sign. Diagnosis of chronic endometritis is made from examining samples of the uterine wall taken with a special biopsy instrument and by examining bacterial swabs. Treatment can vary; antibiotic wash-outs of the uterus are often performed and prostaglandins are used to instigate normal heats.

Vulval Aspiration (Windsucking)

Bad conformation of the vulva can cause a chronic infection of the uterus and thus infertility. The vulval lips should remain closed during all normal movements and should be in an almost vertical position. Sometimes because of damage during foaling, congenital malformation or old age, the natural seal is broken, allowing air to be sucked into the vagina and uterus. Mares that do this are called 'windsuckers'. A chronic infection develops which, as described before, can cause infertility. The treatment applied in these cases is a simple operation called Caslick's operation, which closes the upper portion of the vulval lips and prevents the aspiration of air. Over the next few months the uterus recovers and in many

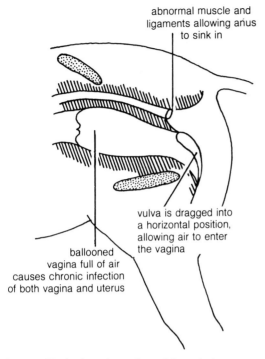

abnormal muscle and ligaments allowing anus to sink in

vulva is dragged into a horizontal position, allowing air to enter the vagina

ballooned vagina full of air causes chronic infection of both vagina and uterus

Fig 34 Typical conformation of the wind-sucking mare.

cases the mare becomes fertile.

The many reasons why your mare might not breed can take some unravelling and it should be stressed that detailed examination by your veterinary surgeon is essential if you want to get your mare in foal or are finding it difficult to do so. Remember too that although the oestrous cycle and a successful ovulation is a very complicated process, the factors that influence it are simple: *the environmental threshold*, involving increased light and warmth, body condition and adequate food.

PREGNANCY DIAGNOSIS

If all fertility problems are over and conception has occurred, it is nice to confirm that a foetus is present to avoid disappointment.

There are three ways of doing this. The traditional way is to ask a veterinary surgeon to examine the mare internally. By feeling the swelling in one of the horns of the uterus, pregnancy can be confirmed. This is usually done from 42 days; however, the more experienced a practitioner, the earlier and more accurately this diagnosis can be made.

The second method relies on the fact that the hormone levels circulating through the body during pregnancy are different from those circulating in an empty, cycling mare. In early pregnancy the level of a hormone called PMSG is high, and later on the oestrogen levels rise. Between 40 and 100 days a test can be carried out on a blood sample to detect PMSG. If this is present, the mare is likely to be pregnant. As pregnancy advances this test becomes unreliable and between 150 and 300 days a test for oestrogens, carried out on a urine sample, is more reliable. Recently a test to detect progesterone in milk or blood has been developed. Using this test we can find out whether progesterone levels are high 19 to 21 days after service. If they are, it is probable that the mare is pregnant.

For those wanting an early, accurate diagnosis, ultrasound is the answer. This machine uses a pulse of high-frequency sound to contrast the organs of the abdomen and to show them on a screen. The sound pulses are generated from a probe which is placed in the mare's rectum. The fluid-filled uterus shows up as a dark shadow with the developing embryo highlighted inside. The advantage of this system is that pregnancy can be demonstrated from 20 days or less with a high degree of accuracy and, more importantly, twins can be detected at an early stage, thus allowing more time for corrective measures to be taken before it becomes too late.

ABORTION

Unfortunately a positive test for pregnancy does not always mean that a foal will be born in eleven months' time. Quite commonly in

Thoroughbred mares, less so in other breeds, abortion occurs. Abortion, or the birth of the foal before 300 days, can be classified in many ways but conveniently we can divide it into abortion due to a non-infective reason and abortion caused by infective agents.

Non-infective

Twins are the most common reason for non-infective abortion. The mare finds it rather difficult to support twins and all too often one of the pair finds that its share of the uterus is not sufficient to support growth. At some time, it gives up the unequal struggle and dies. The other more fortunate twin carries on for a little time, sometimes to full term, but more often it also dies and both are aborted.

The umbilical cord, so important to the health of the foetus, is sometimes too long. When this happens, the chances of it twisting too much are greatly increased and the blood supply to the foal is then interrupted. This causes death of the foal and abortion.

Congenital abnormalities of the embryo are another cause of non-infective abortion.

Infective

The first sign one sees of an infective abortion is generally a small, unhealthy foetus lying on the floor, often surrounded by a thickened diseased placenta. A fungus is the common pathogen involved and infection can occur if the mother eats mouldy hay or, more commonly if the uterus is contaminated at the time of the previous birth. Bacterial infection, again commonly at service, can also cause abortion. Fungal infection generally causes abortion in later pregnancy, and bacterial infection during early pregnancy.

As we have already discussed, another cause of abortion is that caused by the virus Equid herpes type 1. This virus spreads rapidly through a susceptible population and when it infects a pregnant mare it enters the body of the foetus and damages the internal organs, especially the liver and kidneys. Death of the foal follows rapidly and abortion occurs. Infection of the nearly full term foal results in a stillbirth or the delivery of a weak, sickly foal that does not survive long.

NORMAL PREGNANCY AND FOALING

The length of time a mare is normally pregnant – the gestation period – varies between 320 and 380 days. Most mares, however, foal down about 340 days from conception. The foetus in this time grows from a single cell at conception to, at birth, a foal about 34kg in weight; this will be lighter in the pony breeds and heavier in larger working horses. During this time there is very little change. The abdomen of the mare gets larger and, towards the end of gestation, the udder becomes swollen and firm.

Very often the first indication that a mare is about to foal is the presence of a wet, shaky foal, trying very hard to rise to its feet and get to mother and the milk bank. However, there are a few clues that birth is imminent. The enlargement of the mammary glands (udder) accelerates and waxing, a honey-coloured secretion which forms at the end of each teat, occurs. The composition of the colostrum – the first milk – also changes just before foaling. The level of calcium, sodium and potassium salts becomes higher. By measuring the concentration of these salts, the time of birth can be estimated within 24 hours. Other physical changes occur: the pelvic ligaments become softer and the musculature around the anus and vagina slackens. The behaviour of the mare changes. At first she becomes antisocial, then nervous. Unfortunately the margin of error is wide and these signs can occur several times before foaling actually starts.

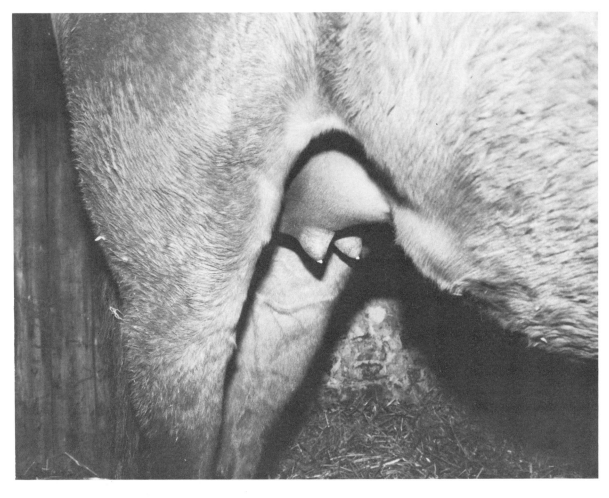

Fig 35   The full mammary gland and 'waxing' indicate that the mare is near to term.

Labour

If one is lucky enough actually to observe a mare foaling, the first signs could easily be confused with colic, that is, discomfort, sweating and frequent passing of faeces and urine. This signifies the start of the first stage. For convenience labour can be divided into three stages.

First stage   The first stage begins when the uterus starts its first waves of contraction. These periods of contraction are spasmodic to begin with and the mare frequently becomes relaxed enough to wander around the box, perhaps to eat some hay, before another wave starts off another bout of discomfort. Some mares seem hardly bothered at all but others, generally younger mothers, can become very disturbed. As the intensity of contractions builds up, the cervix gradually opens and the uterine pressure forces the foetal membranes into the vagina. When these rupture, releasing ten to twenty litres of fluid, a process known as 'breaking of the waters', the second stage of labour, can be said to have started.

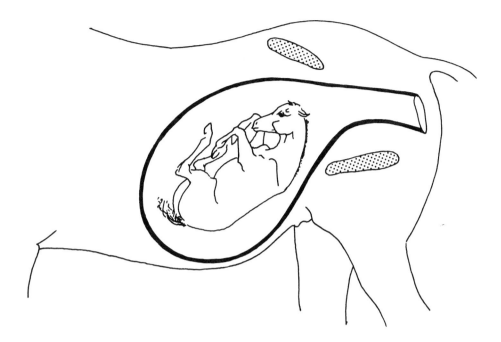

Fig 36   The normal position of the foal before parturition.

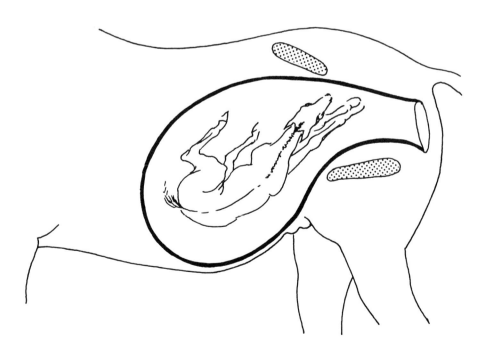

Fig 37   During the first stage of labour, the foal twists so that the head
and forelimbs are in a dorsal position.

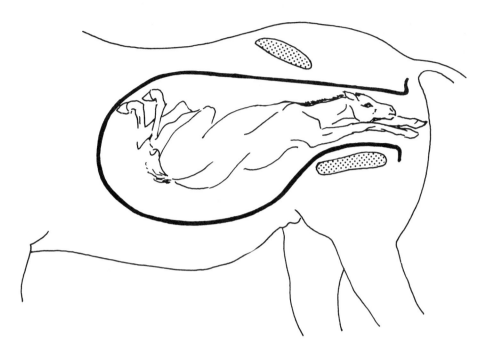

Fig 38　During the second stage, the foal's head and chest are presented in the dorsal position. The hind quarters, however, are still lying ventrally.

Second stage　If possible, the time that the waters break should be noted, as from this point labour is irreversible and should only take 40 minutes, less in some mares. The mare lies down and starts to strain; on her side she finds it easier to push the foal into the pelvic girdle. At first she gets up and down several times, possibly to help to reposition the foal. In late pregnancy the foal lies on its back with legs folded to its belly, then during the first stage of labour the foal twists so that the head and chest are now the right way up and the front legs extend into the pelvic canal. How this is managed is not understood, but the frequent getting up and down of the mare, the contractions of the uterus and the foal's own movements are all involved.

By now the mare is working quite hard. First a shiny membrane appears at the vulva. This, the amnion, is the membrane which surrounds the foal. Then the front feet can be seen, one just before the other, followed shortly by the nose, head and chest of the foal. It is at this stage that the foal's movements break the amnion. If this does not happen, the membranes should be broken to free the foal and allow him to breathe. The whole process is fast and violent, taking five to fifteen minutes only. After a short rest, one last effort produces the foal's hips and hind quarters and the foal is delivered.

It is now that the mare should not be disturbed, as a sudden rise to her feet could break the cord and hence jeopardise the foal's life because during this period of rest the blood remaining in the placental membranes is pumped into the foal's system. The loss of this quantity of blood could make the difference between survival and death of the new-born foal. The hind legs often lie in the vaginal passage for a few minutes. This is perhaps nature's way of plugging a potential gateway by which infections could enter the uterus. Now the mare rises to her feet to turn and

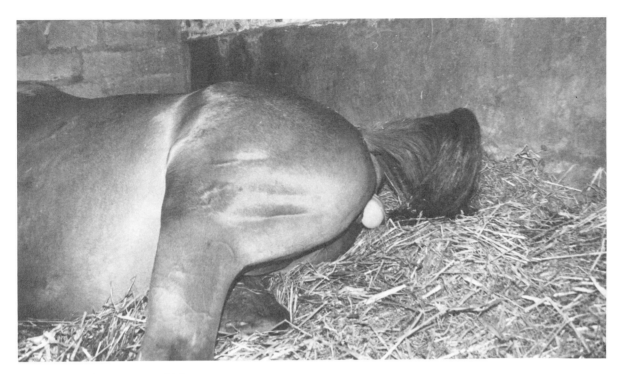

Fig 39   Early in stage two of labour.

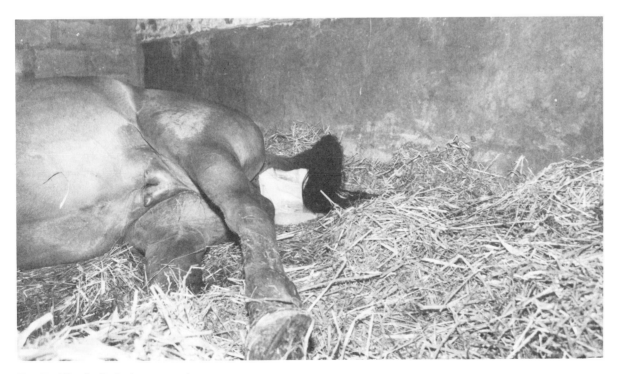

Fig 40   The foal's feet can now be seen.

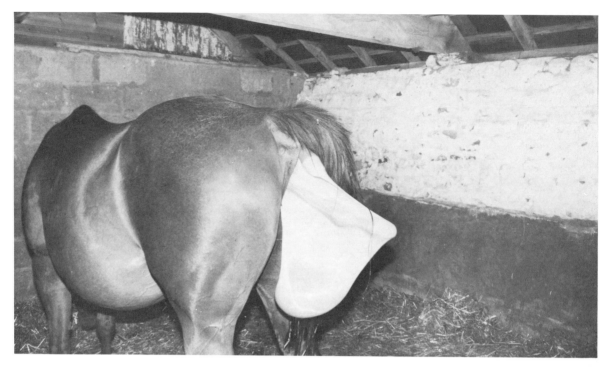

Fig 41 The mare gets up, probably to change the foal's position.

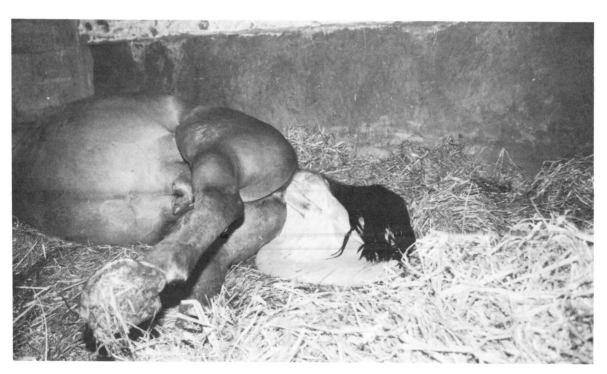

Fig 42 Now the head is presented.

74

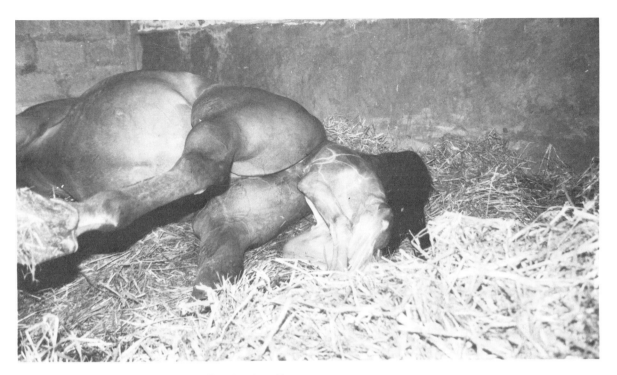

Fig 43   Things happen quickly now. The foal is half out.

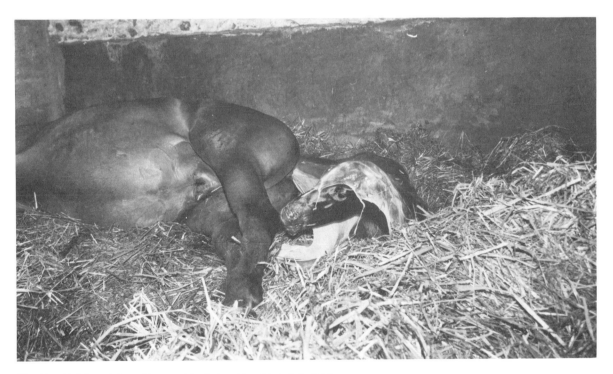

Fig 44   At this point, mother and foal should not be disturbed.

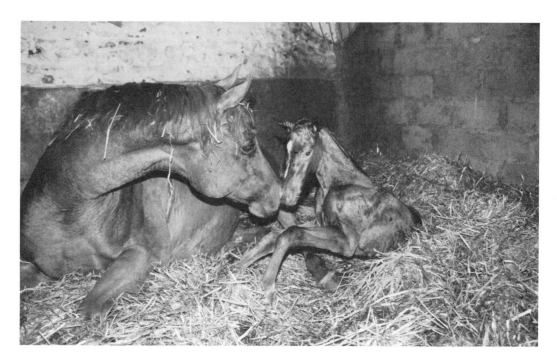

Fig 45   Getting acquainted.

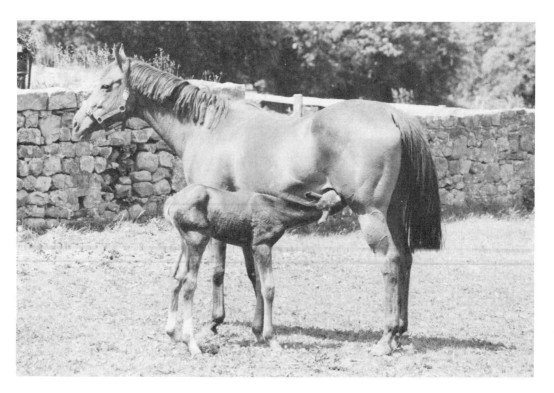

Fig 46   The next day.

inspect the new arrival and to start the cleansing process. This action imprints the image of mother in the foal's mind and stimulates the reflexes necessary to cope with the outside world. During the resting period another vital change takes place – the umbilical cord becomes brittle. This allows either the foal's movements, or the mother rising, to break the correct place, about 3.25cm from the abdomen. This physical change occurs in order to minimise the chances of infection entering via the cord, or haemorrhage occurring from the stump. All that needs to be done at this time is to treat the end of the cord with an antibacterial powder or solution.

What can go wrong at this stage? Fortunately very little. However, if anything should, it must be treated as an emergency. If the foal has not arrived within twenty minutes of strong contractions, get in touch with your veterinary surgeon immediately as a wasted journey is much better than a dead foal or a damaged mother.

Third stage The third stage of labour takes place about an hour after the birth of the foal. During this stage the afterbirth – the placenta – is expelled and the uterus starts to contract to its non-pregnant size. Don't worry about the slight signs of colic shown at this time – these are quite normal. Once the placenta has been dropped, it should be spread out and examined to check whether it is all there, as any bits left in the uterus could cause acute endometritis – infection of the uterus – and the risk of other diseases such as laminitis. If the placenta has not been dropped within six hours, your vet should be consulted. He will probably remove it manually and treat the mare, to minimise any risk of infection. The appearance of the placenta should also be noticed, and any diseased, thickened bits should be kept and shown to your veterinary surgeon, since they may indicate a diseased uterus and possible damage to the foal.

DISEASES OF THE FOAL

The most important thing the new-born foal does, once it has struggled to its feet, is to search under its mother's belly for the udder and its first feed. It is essential that this feed of colostrum is safely in the foal's stomach within a few hours of birth. If not, the all-important antibodies which the mother's colostrum contains will not be absorbed into the body. The immunity they give to the foal will protect it through the vital first few months of life and without adequate levels, neonatal disease becomes a serious threat to its life. So, if the foal has not fed in the first few hours, try and persuade him to suck; failing this, milk the mare and feed him by hand. Don't, however, go overboard with the attention. Remember that the newborn foal is severely stressed. Give it time to recover from the birth trauma before fussing. Attention which is too early might also confuse it and before you know it, the foal will have adopted you as its mother. Once this has happened, to persuade it otherwise is a difficult task.

Foal Septicaemia

Foal septicaemia is one disease that commonly affects the colostrum-deprived foal. Sometimes the causal organism can infect the foal whilst it is still in the uterus or, more commonly, it enters the umbilical stump at or soon after birth. The disease can be acute, causing death in the first twenty-four hours, but more often it causes a subacute disease lasting four to seven days. Swelling of the joints, enteritis and abscess formation in the lungs and kidneys are the usual sequelae.

Treatment must be immediate, as any delay will allow the organisms responsible to cause lesions in joint and lung which are difficult to cure. The practice of administering routine antibiotics after birth may help to prevent septicaemia, as will prompt dressing of the umbilical stump with an antiseptic solution.

Foaling boxes must be thoroughly cleansed and disinfected after each foaling.

Infective Arthritis (Joint Ill)

This disease occurs at any time between birth and 3 months of age. It is a common sequel to septicaemia but it can also exist as a separate entity. Lameness in one or more limbs, generally with swelling of the affected joint, is the first sign noticed. The joint becomes hot and painful, the body temperature rises to between 102 and 104F and the foal stops sucking.

Very often the state of the mare's udder gives a better indication of the foal's health than the foal itself. Always check a foal carefully if the mother's udder is swollen, or if milk is escaping from the teat, as this generally means that the foal is ill.

As with many foal diseases, it is essential to start treatment of joint ill as soon as any signs are seen. Any delay and the damage done to the joint surfaces and the bone will be irreparable. A long course of an effective antibiotic, given early in the disease, will sometimes but not always cure the condition.

Retained Meconium

Colt foals – especially large ones – sometimes find it difficult to pass the meconium, the name given to the faeces which have collected in the rectum during pregnancy. Normally meconium is passed within a few hours of birth. It can be recognised by its colour, a greeny brown, and is quickly followed by normal milk faeces which are orange-yellow in colour. The first signs of meconium retention are colicky in nature. The tail starts twitching, the foal keeps on straining and discomfort gradually increases in intensity. Very quickly the foal loses interest in sucking and spends much time lying down. The head is frequently lifted to inspect the flank, a sure sign of gut pain. If left untreated, peritonitis – infection of the lining of the abdomen – rapidly intervenes and the foal becomes critically ill. This condition is potentially very serious so watch your foal carefully until all the meconium has been passed. The colour change as normal milk faeces come through will tell you when this has occurred.

Removing the mass of meconium is a job for the experienced. A combination of oral liquid paraffin and enemas will move most blockages but as a last resort surgery has to be performed. Again, any delay in seeking professional help is dangerous.

Foal Enteritis (Diarrhoea)

Enteritis is common in the young foal. The mare often comes into heat eight or so days after foaling and the hormones responsible for heat – oestrogens – which are present in the milk, can cause diarrhoea in the foal. As long as the foal looks well and keeps on feeding then little harm is done and no treatment is needed. In these cases, a little common sense is needed. Does the foal look ill? If it does, call your vet.

Sometimes the diarrhoea does not get better, or the foal is infected by bacteria which cause severe enteritis. *E coli* and *Salmonella* species are among the common culprits. It is important to realise that it is the loss of fluid from the foal's system that does most of the harm. The dehydration caused by the loss of fluid, and the fever caused by the bacteria, stop the foal sucking and thus make the dehydration worse. In these cases it is more important to correct the dehydration than to treat the enteritis. This is done by administering electrolyte fluids — a mixture of salts and water approximating to the composition of the foal's own body fluids — by mouth, or in more serious cases, by intravenous injection, directly into the blood. Effective antibiotics should be given to control the infection.

Haemolytic Disease

In the non-thoroughbred this is rather a rare disease of the new-born foal affecting the blood system. The red blood cells of the infant are destroyed by antibodies which the foal absorbs from its mother's colostrum. The antibodies are formed by the mother in response to the small amounts of foal's blood which leak into her system through the placental barrier. Some mothers assume that this is foreign material and antibodies are formed to combat the mistaken threat. The destruction of large numbers of the foal's red blood cells causes a severe anaemia and the waste products produce a jaundice.

The symptoms of haemolytic disease occur within 48 hours of birth. The first signs are rapid breathing and an accelerated heart beat, due to the anaemia, and yellowing of the whites of the eyes and mucous membranes due to jaundice. Blood-stained urine is frequently present. The treatment consists of removing the foal from the source of the problem, the colostrum, and transfusing the foal with a new blood supply. Once a mare has generated these antibodies she is likely to do so again in subsequent foalings and future foals should be removed from the mare and given colostrum from another mare for the first 48 hours.

Parasitic Diseases

As the foal gets older the two common worms affecting foals can cause trouble. *Strongyloides westeri* is found in the younger foal, two to four months old. *Parascaris Equorum* – the large white worm – causes trouble in older foals. (*See* Chapter 4)

Physical Abnormalities

As soon as possible after the foal is born, you should give it a close examination to check whether there are any abnormalities present.

One group of abnormalities which are immediately apparent, the angular limb deformities, are dealt with later (*see* Chapter 10). Other physical abnormalities which are commonly seen are ruptures and hernias. In such cases the body wall is absent or so damaged that the contents of the abdomen escape and lie under the skin. Two common sites of herniation are the umbilicus and in the male, the inguinal ring. Hernias should be examined by a veterinary surgeon without delay, when a decision can be made whether the defect needs immediate repair.

Accidents

By far the most common reason for veterinary attention to the young foal is an accident. Young foals are excitable, very fit and can travel at great speed. In the wrong environment this can be a recipe for disaster. Remove all barbed wire, all sheets of tin and round out sharp corners. Even taking these precautions, your foal is likely to get cut, so vaccinate against tetanus as soon as possible.

Routine Procedures

Although neither an illness nor a surgical treatment, castration of the colt deserves a few words.

Castration is the surgical removal of both testicles from the male horse. The reasons for doing so are firstly to render the colt infertile, and secondly to remove the socially unwanted aspects of male behaviour. The operation can be performed at any age, but it is most usual to castrate a colt when he is between one and two years of age. The traditional time to operate is either the spring or autumn, both periods when the number of flies is minimal and the risk of post-operative infection at its lowest.

The operation can be carried out in the tanding position, under local anaesthesia, ith the colt sedated. However, the safety of both surgeon and patient would be better served using general anaesthesia. Nowadays most veterinary surgeons operate on the recumbent colt under general anaesthesia. In this manner, the operation can be carried out calmly, with good visibility and plenty of time to ensure that all the testicular tissue is removed.

Rigs (Cryptorchids)

Occasionally a colt has one or both testicles missing. In such cases, the testicles are present but have not descended through the inguinal ring into the scrotum. These colts are called rigs (cryptorchids) and they pose a problem. If the visible testicle is removed, the testicle that is hidden in the ring or in the abdomen is still able to secrete male hormones and a horse that appears to be a gelding acts like a stallion.

In these cases, the veterinary surgeon first explores the ring from the outside in an attempt to find the testicle. If he does so, the testicle can be gently exteriorised and removed; if not, a major abdominal operation is necessary to find and remove the undescended testicle.

Some horses display stallion characteristics even though no testicular tissue can be found in their body and no male hormones demonstrated in the blood. A laboratory test can be carried out which, by measuring testosterone levels, identifies these 'false rigs'. No reason for this behaviour has been found, but it appears most often when a strange horse is introduced into a field of mares. The antisocial behaviour usually dies down after a few months.

8 Ocular and Auditory Systems

THE EYE

The eye of the horse is an organ which, until recently, has received little scientific attention. It is not easily studied without specialised equipment, although much can be gained from careful observation, coupled with the use of a pen torch and a hand-held lens. Furthermore, treatment can create more damage when not carefully and correctly undertaken.

Anatomy and Physiology

The eye can be likened in structure and function to a complex camera: light is received through the transparent cornea and passes through a variable light diaphragm, the iris, before the parallel light waves are focused by the lens on to the light-sensitive retina which lines the inside of the back of the eye – the fundus. The retina converts the light signal into an electrical signal by way of a chemical change in pigment, and then transmits the electrical wave through the optic nerve to the brain. Eyelids serve to protect the delicate structures of the eye from damage from the external environment. A membrane called the conjunctiva runs over the surface of the cornea and is reflected back inside the eyelids.

The retina is an extension of the brain, protected by a tough, fibrous coat – the sclera – which obtains its nutrition from the uvea (the middle coat, or layer, of the eyeball). The sclera (the eye's white, outer covering) becomes transparent cornea at the front. The cornea is completely devoid of blood vessels but extremely sensitive to pain and touch. The eye's shape is kept by fluid pressure from within. The lens is attached by extensions of the uvea which have a limited ability to alter the shape of the lens to allow focusing on near or distant objects. It separates the clear, liquid aqueous humour in front from the clear, jelly-like vitreous humour behind.

Part of the uvea extends as a choroid containing many blood vessels and lining the fundus outside the retina. Within the choroid is a layer known as the tapetum which is heavily pigmented and reflects the light that has passed through the retina back through the retina, so that vision is increased, particularly where the light intensity is low.

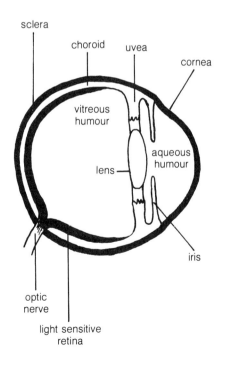

Fig 47 Section through the horse's eye.

The iris acts as an aperture which reduces in size in bright light to control the amount of light passing to the retina. The iris is oval in shape and irregular in outline, due to black projections from the margins into the aperture. These projections (corpora nigra) may obstruct vision to a limited extent in bright light, when the pupil is constricted. The corpora nigra are thought to reduce the glare of bright light. In the camel, which is subject to much more glare, they are more developed.

Occasionally larger tadpole-like cysts may be attached to the iris. They vary in size according to the degree of dilation of the pupil, but do not affect vision.

'Wall' or 'China' eye refers to an eye in which the colour of the iris is white. This is of no significance except on rare occasions when it is associated with inflammation. The condition is more common in older horses.

Due to a complex series of muscle attachments, the eye can be moved freely in many directions within the orbit, but even without movement the horse's field of vision in the horizontal plane covers approximately 320

degrees; in the vertical plane it is 178 degrees. This is because the eyes are placed at the sides of the head. As a result, the area covered by vision with *both* eyes, stereoscopic vision, is limited.

Tears are produced in the lacrimal gland between the upper, outer margin of the eye and the overlying bone. Their function is to keep the surface of the eye moist. They are used in conjunction with the eyelids to wipe away dust and debris. The fluid drains into the inner corner of the eye, where it passes down the nasolacrimal duct and into the nostril. Careful observation will reveal a small hole just inside the horse's nostril which indicates the duct's site of exit.

A cartilaginous third eyelid known as the nictitating membrane normally lies on the lower margin of the eye, inside the lower eyelid and towards the nose. On occasions it can be raised and brought across the lower half of the eye.

Examination

The purpose of examining the eye is to detect whether any abnormality is present. If one is present, we must ask whether:

1. it is likely to affect the horse's vision
2. it is likely to be progressive
3. it is likely to recur
4. it can be treated.

When the examination is being made on behalf of a potential purchaser, he is interested only in the first three. Where a condition is present but does not affect vision and is not likely to progress or recur it is simply noted as a blemish. A horse with only one eye can still be suitable for some work provided that it is not likely to meet unexpected challenges or have to work at speed.

Much can be learned from a look at the size of one eye compared with its opposite, the position of the eye (whether it is shrunken

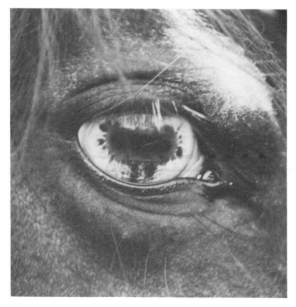

Fig 48 Wall eye.

back or protruding, for example), and from determining whether there is discharge from the eye, loss of tears (lacrimation) or swelling around the eye. Before handling, it is often valuable to take swabs or scrapings from the conjunctiva, for isolation of bacteria or fungi. Fungi are very slow growing and a month should be allowed before growth can be considered negative.

By shining a beam of light into the eye, the outer structures can be more easily seen. The lens often looks quite opaque in bright light. The ability of the retina to receive light and respond can be tested, since when a bright light is shone into one eye, both pupils should constrict rapidly. Failure to respond suggests either an obstruction between the light source and the light-sensitive retina, or damage to the nervous system of the eye.

To examine the deeper structures of the eye, an ophthalmoscope is needed, usually a direct ophthalmoscope which magnifies and focuses the structures of the eye, particularly the iris, the lens, the vitreous humour and the retina. Occasionally a yellow stain – fluorescein – is used on the surface of the eye. Irregularities such as ulceration causing damage to the cornea will become highlighted as a green stain.

Examination of the eye is not always easy. Frequently, particularly in foals, the use of sedatives to restrain the animal is very valuable, particularly during treatment. Application of local anaesthetic to the surface of the eye is also helpful. However, more extensive treatment or interference within the eye requires general anaesthesia.

When a lesion is found in the eye the horse's vision may need to be assessed, which can be done by placing the animal in an unusual environment and asking it to follow a course in which small obstacles have been placed.

Treatment

It is normal, where possible, to avoid surgical interference with the eye, since such surgery is automatically very delicate and the chances of complications are high. However, surgery is becoming more readily considered in treatment. Minor procedures in particular can be used, such as the placing of a tube temporarily into the eye, through which regular treatment can be passed without handling the eye itself. The eyelids can then be sutured together to provide support and protection to the cornea, aiding healing. Where damage to the eye is very severe, unpleasant to look at and unlikely to repair sufficiently for sight to be restored, it is possible to remove the eye. One frequently unacceptable result is that the orbital cavity is left, lined with skin. It is now possible to place a silicon implant into the orbit so that the skin is tight across the eye socket. The resulting effect is cosmetically much more pleasant.

In the United States, surgery purely for cosmetic purposes is becoming more common. Contact lenses are regularly fitted to valuable show animals whose corneas have been badly scarred. A cosmetic shell may be placed over the top of a chronically shrunken eye which has sustained severe damage, in an effort to supply two identically sized (and marked) eyes. Surgery for cosmetics reasons, however, raises a number of moral and ethical considerations.

DISEASE OF THE EYE

Globe

Occasionally one or both eyes are too small. This may be a congenital problem, and when this happens there may also be the presence of cataracts and/or defects of the iris or retina. No treatment is available in these cases.

Shrinkage of the eye (phthisis bulbi) may be the final stage following severe damage to the eye. Again, corrective treatment is not possible at this stage.

Bulging of the eye (exophthalmus), without any apparent abnormality within the eye, often results from something behind the eye putting pressure on the globe. Either an abscess, following infection, or a growth (tumour) may be the cause, but in the latter case, the rate of onset of exophthalmus is usually slower.

Eyelids

Entropion is a condition affecting one or both eyes of the new-born foal; the eyelids roll in, so that the hairs on the outer surfaces of the eyelids rub on the cornea, causing irritation. Excessively long eyelids or shrinkage of the eye into the orbit may be causes. Normally temporary turning out again, using stitches, is adequate to correct the problem, but occasionally a small piece of skin must be taken from the eyelid to shorten it.

The opposite condition, ectropion, in which the eyelids are turned out, can occur but is rare.

Neoplasia, or growth formations, frequently occur around the eye. The most common type

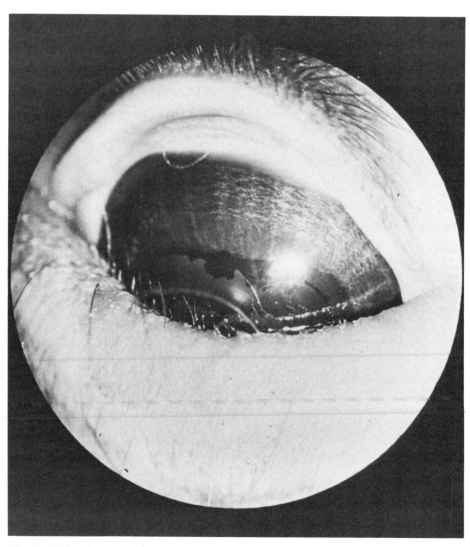

Fig 49   Entropion

is the sarcoid, which usually occurs at multiple sites on the skin. Removal by cutting away from the site can be difficult and the most successful treatment currently available is to remove the bulk of the growth and freeze what is left to destroy the tissue. The dead tissue will then slough over ten to fourteen days. If all the neoplastic tissue is removed, the growth will not generally recur. A few tumours, particularly on greys, have the potential to be highly malignant, spreading rapidly.

It should be remembered that the most diagnostic sign of tetanus is spasm of the third eyelid. However, this is part of a much wider clinical picture (*see* Chapter 11).

Conjunctiva

Occasionally foals are born with skin-like tissue, including hair, in an abnormal site, either on the cornea or on the conjunctiva as it runs over the eyeball. By careful cutting, the tissue can be surgically removed.

Conjunctivitis causing inflammation and reddening around the eye is uncommon in the horse. A variety of types of organisms may be involved, either as a primary infection, or secondary to physical damage to the conjunctiva. Although bacteria are most frequently implicated, parasites, viruses and, in the tropics, even fungi may cause damage. Treatment needs to be directed towards the specific cause.

Growths or tumours are not uncommon on the conjunctiva, the most common again being sarcoids but squamous cell carcinomas (cancers) also occur where horses are exposed to bright sunlight, and malignant melanomas in grey horses. All such tumours are potentially very serious because they invade local tissue and are very difficult to remove completely. They may also spread to other sites.

Cornea

Perhaps the most vulnerable part of the eye is the cornea and it is not surprising that physical damage to it is probably the most common eye problem encountered. Usually an area of the surface of the cornea is lost, affecting a variable depth and producing an ulcer. The eyelids are pressed tightly together and tears run down the outside of the face. The horse shows obvious pain which is made worse by bright light. The same picture is seen following corneal infection, which is usually a sequel to traumatic injury.

The surface of the eye has a very poor blood supply since blood vessels in this area would impair vision. Consequently, when the tissues are damaged, the cornea becomes very vulnerable to secondary infection with bacteria or fungi, which rapidly cause further damage. Repair of the damaged cornea is brought about by blood vessels moving from the edge of the cornea nearest to the site of injury, and growing to the site. Until this blood supply has become established (after which healing is usually rapid) it is important to prevent infection, by regularly instilling antibiotic and antifungal agents into the eye, up to six times daily. It is also vital to avoid using corticosteroids in the eye, since these will slow the rate of healing, allowing organisms to cause damage which may result in complete erosion of the cornea and its perforation. Since many eye ointment preparations contain corticosteroids, any which are left after a prescribed course of treatment should be discarded to avoid the temptation of using them subsequently without qualified advice. Antibiotics and other drugs are often injected under the conjunctiva where they are slowly released into surrounding tissues to give a high local concentration.

Lacerations on the cornea can be stitched using usually very fine silk and this reduces the ultimate scarring. Scarring is *usually* slight and has little effect on vision; however, the effect that scarring has on vision must be judged in each individual case. Where the cornea is completely perforated, the fluid centre of the eye is lost and the iris may also come through the perforation, sealing the wound but often causing bleeding into the eye in the process.

The cornea can also be affected by viruses, particularly Equine Herpes Virus, producing puncture-like damage to the cornea.

Yeasts and fungi are fairly common as causes of infection. They need prolonged periods of treatment. Response to treatment is generally not good and where infection spreads into the eye, the eye will be lost.

Uvea

The anterior uvea consists of the structures which support the lens, namely the iris and the ciliary body. Inflammation of the uvea (uveitis) produces obvious pain, tight shutting of the eyelids and constriction of the pupil. Cloudy material may appear behind the cor-

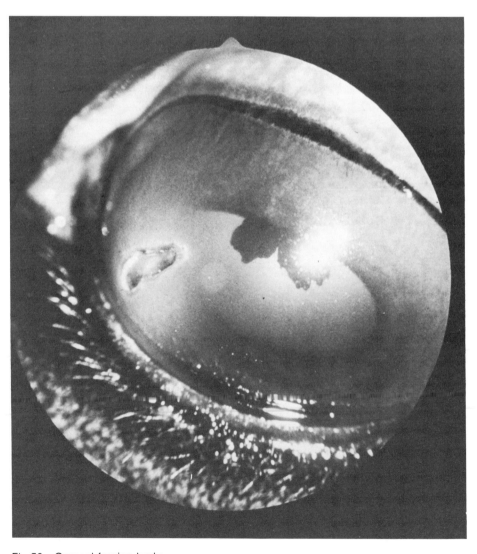

Fig 50   Corneal foreign body

nea. In the later stages, material may deposit on the lens surface with rough pitting of the lens and cloudiness (cataract) within the lens. The iris may stick to the lens so that the pupil cannot dilate or constrict properly.

Uveitis is the response to a variety of assaults. It may be a reflex response after damage to the cornea, or after traumatic injury, particularly if infection is introduced. However, infection by a variety of bacteria and viruses may obtain access through the blood supply. Most frequently, though, the cause is unknown. In these cases the condition usually affects only one eye and often recurs, hence the name 'Periodic Ophthalmia', or 'Moon Blindness', since recurrence appears to be in phase with the moon. Thoroughbreds of two to three years are most commonly affected. Treatment with anti-inflammatory agents must be intense and prolonged if any success is likely. Various factors have been blamed. In the United States certain bacteria (*Leptospira*

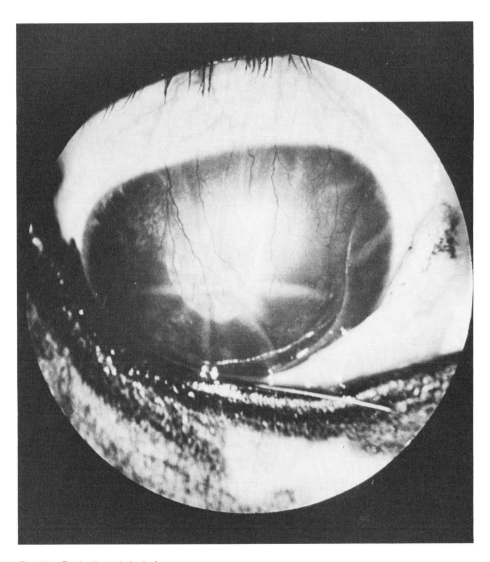

Fig 51   Periodic ophthalmia

pomona) are accepted to be the cause. In Britain worms (*onchocerca*), bacteria, viruses, vitamin B deficiency in the diet and allergy to an unknown substance have all been postulated as causes. Currently the cause is accepted to be an immune response by the horse to a wide variety of organisms.

Lens

Although in the horse the lens is not as important as it is in man, abnormalities can seriously affect vision. Any opacity in the lens or its capsule is defined as a cataract.

Cataracts are often confused with concentric rings in the lens which indicate irregular development. When examined through the ophthalmoscope these rings resemble onion rings. The retina at the back of the eye can easily be seen through them and they are of no consequence.

True cataracts have a variety of origins. In foals under a year old they will probably be congenital, that is, the foal is born with them.

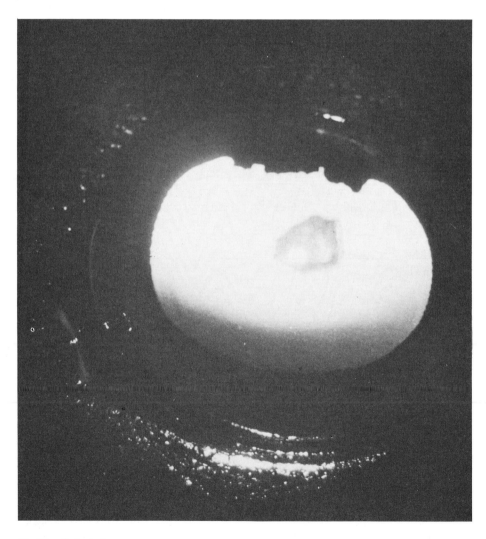

Fig 52   Cataract

One or both eyes may be affected to a degree, varying from a small point of opacity to (more often) a totally diffuse area causing complete blindness in that eye. Functional vision may be partially restored by removing badly affected lenses, a procedure which is most effective if performed before six months of age.

Senile cataracts, similar to those which occur in old dogs are rare in horses. Where cataracts occur later in life they may be a sequel to periodic ophthalmia or any other form of uveitis, as has already been discussed, or as a result of trauma such as a fall during racing or jumping. Where cataracts due to trauma generally occur on the front of the lens and are not progressive, those that follow uveitis usually show an increase in density of the fibres of the lens, with a cobweb-like or granular appearance through the ophthalmoscope, and these are progressive.

Any cataract which is found on examination may either increase in size and density with time, or may remain or reduce. Which line the opacity will follow is almost impossible to predict from a single examination, so it is prudent to err on the side of caution and assume that the condition will deteriorate until evidence proves otherwise.

THE EARS

The horse has a well-developed sense of hearing, enabling him to hear sounds from up to 4.4 km away although, in common with humans, his ability to hear high frequencies decreases with age. One reason for his keen hearing ability is that the cartilagenous pinna (the visible, external part of the ear) is funnel shaped to catch the sound. Ten muscles at the base allow the ear to be turned to locate sound accurately. Man has only three muscles, and these are very poorly developed.

Most ear problems relate to the pinna. The large, white aural plaques on the inside of the pinna and tumours, particularly sarcoids, on the outside are covered in Chapter 9.

Damage to the pinna, causing tearing of the cartilage, may be slow to heal and stitching of the ear needs to be done in two or more separate layers.

Occasionally in young horses a large swelling may be present at the base of the ear, producing a persistent discharge. If this dentigerous ('tooth bearing') cyst is removed surgically, as it will need to be if the discharge is to be stopped, it will be found to contain greasy sebaceous material, possibly with hair and tooth material.

At the bottom of the vertical canal going down inside the ear, there is a 90 degree turn where the canal goes into bone. Here it acts as the short, external auditory meatus (canal connecting the external opening with the ear drum) which terminates in the drum. The horizontal canal may become inhabited by ear mites of the genus *Psoroptes*. Infested horses often become head-shy when handled around the ears, rub their ears when allowed to, and make sudden, abnormal head movements when ridden. Diagnosis is difficult to confirm since general anaesthesia is needed to penetrate this far into the ear canal. However, 0.01 per cent gamma BHC is very effective in killing the mites.

Because of its very protected position, the ear drum very rarely becomes damaged. The middle ear has a series of three bones – the mallus, incus and stapes – which act to amplify the sound on the ear drum. A tube – *the Eustachian tube* – extends from the middle ear cavity to the throat, allowing pressure on each side of the ear drum to be equalized. The guttural pouches are two large sacs leading off the Eustachian tubes.

The middle ear is separated from the inner ear by a membrane. The inner ear is a membranous labyrinth in a sealed, fluid-filled bag. A vestibule has a cochlear duct running inside a coiled cochlea, which is responsible for hearing, together with three semicircular ducts in canals set at right angles to each other, in three

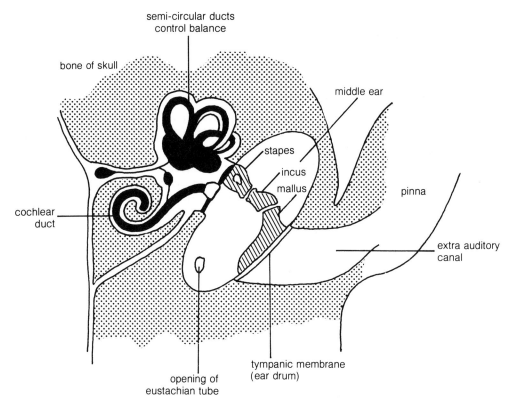

Fig 53 Section through the horse's ear.

dimensions, which control movement and balance.

Damage to the inner ear is extremely unlikely in the horse but may result from a severe blow on the head, causing bleeding within the inner ear, or extension of infection from the external auditory meatus across the middle ear and into the inner ear. Both situations will be revealed by incoordination in movement and balance, usually with a head tilt.

9　The Skin

The diseases of the skin provide a considerable proportion of the cases that veterinary surgeons see and treat during their working week. Their immediate visibility means that the concerned horseman notices the condition quickly and seeks professional help without delay. However, the low mortality of most skin diseases often tempts the 'do it yourself' merchant to try out a bewildering array of potions and creams before seeking professional help. This makes an accurate diagnosis all the more difficult, as the original lesions are often unrecognisable.

The skin fulfils a whole set of functions that we perhaps take for granted. Together with the hair and the sweat glands, it helps to keep the body temperature constant. Its varying thickness at different parts of the body has an important protective function and the numerous nerves which end in the skin serve to warn the horse of any potentially painful situation.

INFECTIONS

Like any organ, the skin can be infected with bacteria, with fungi or with viruses. The initial damage is seldom serious but the intense irritation that accompanies such lesions may cause the horse to rub them. This self-mutilation quickly increases the area and degree of damage which, in its turn, increases the irritation. This cycle must be broken before any cure can be ensured.

Bacterial Infections

Horses get boils just as we can. In the horse these are generally caused by a bacterium called *staphylococcus*. Small lumps appear in the skin which come to a head and burst, releasing a sticky pus which mats the hairs together. The treatment consists of first bathing the area with hot water, to encourage the abscess to burst, then applying an antibiotic or antiseptic ointment to the area. If there are too many boils to treat individually then a course of an effective antibiotic should be given.

Ringworm

Ringworm in the horse is caused by a group of fungi of which the two most common are called *Trichophyton* and *Microsporum*. The horse is either infected directly from another animal (the ringworm fungus knows no barriers and can infect many species) or can be infected indirectly from contaminated tack, blankets or brushes. As the fungus grows on the skin it produces tiny spores which are spread to other parts of the body by grooming or by the rubbing action of tack or blankets. Here they set up other infected foci which quickly develop into the typical ringworm lesions, round scabby rings in groups along the girth area, under the saddle or along the edge of the rug.

Several successful treatments exist for ringworm; these can be used either individually or together. The antibiotic griseofulvin works well against the *Trichophyton* type of ringworm, less well against *Microsporum* species. The method of treatment is to include the antibiotic in the feed every day for one week. Griseofulvin is concentrated in the skin and prevents the fungus from growing. Another antibiotic called natamycin is active against ringworm and is used as a wash at the site of infection. It is important to cover the whole body to reach the lesions that are not yet

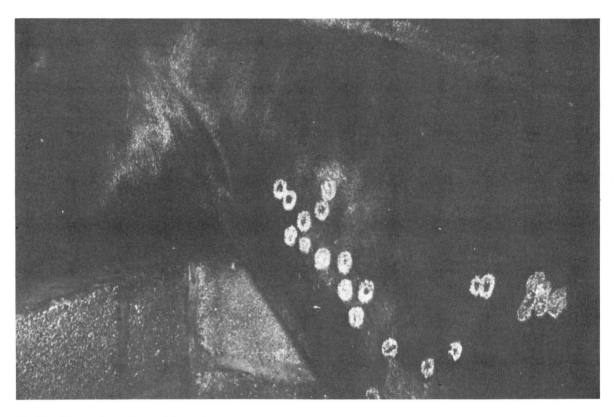

Fig 54   Ringworm at its most typical.

apparent. The treatment must be repeated every fourth day, at least three times.

Dermatophilus Infections

Both mud fever and rain scald are caused by bacteria called *Dermatophilus congolensis*.

Rain scald   As its name suggests, this is a condition that usually develops when the weather is permanently wet, especially when the temperature and humidity are high. The organism multiplies in the warm, damp conditions under the hair and damages the surface of the skin. Large quantities of serum ooze out of the raw skin and mat the hair together, forming areas of crusty scabs. These areas spread as the organism is carried down the body along the natural 'rain run off' pathways, and at its worst this can involve all exposed parts of the body. In the early stages, the disease can best be recognised by running a hand over the body. Small lumps caused by matted hair can be felt deep down close to the skin surface. Microscopic examination of the moist underside of the scab will show the typical branching network of organisms.

Mud fever   This condition is not as dependent on temperature as rain scald, but it does thrive in muddy, wet conditions. The abrasive effect of mud particles on soggy, wet skin opens up small cracks which become infected with *dermatophilus*, and inflamed, swollen lesions quickly develop. The lesions of mud fever first develop on the back of the fetlock area and white legs seem to be more susceptible. If mud fever is untreated it rapidly spreads up the leg to involve the flexor tendons and here can cause a serious infection and an acutely lame horse.

92

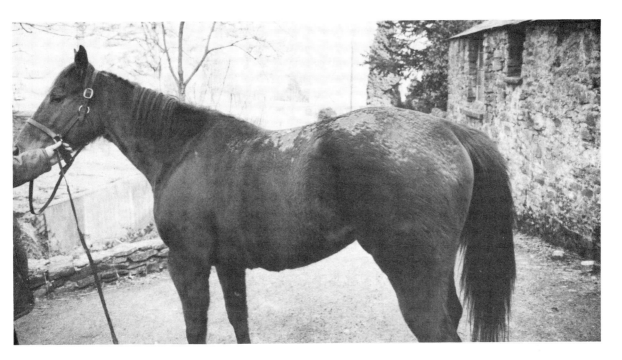

Fig 55   Typical lesions of half-healed rain scald.

Treatment   The treatments for both mud fever and rain scald follow the same pattern. *Dermatophilus* thrives in wet conditions, thus the first and most important stage in the treatment is to keep the horse dry at all times. This is essential. The rain scalded horse will have to be stabled in a well-ventilated box and the horse with mud fever must avoid mud and wet at all costs. Any exercising should be done on dry roads. The scabs of matted hair must be removed by gentle grooming; the immediate appearance will be a lot worse, as large areas of raw, inflamed skin are exposed, but in this way *dermatophilus* loses its favourite wet environment. The application of a mild antiseptic wash should now complete the job. The smaller lesions of mud fever can be treated with a combined cleansing antiseptic lotion. Severe cases of both conditions may need treatment with antibiotics.

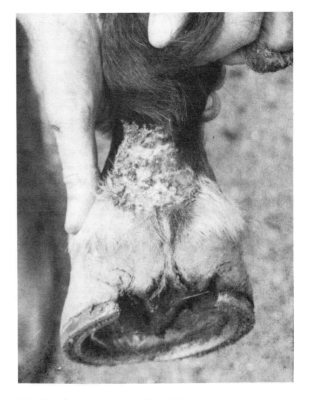

Fig 56   A typical case of mud fever.

PARASITIC DISEASES

Lice

Horse lice – both biting and sucking types – live in the depths of the horse's coat. They are small active creatures about 2 mm long and feed on skin debris and body fluids. The active movement and the intense irritation of their bites causes the horse to rub the affected areas; shoulders and neck are common sites and these rapidly become bald. Severe infestations can cause loss of condition due to anaemia.

During the summer months the numbers of lice are low, but as winter approaches the hair grows longer, horses are kept closer together and the lice start to breed. The eggs, or nits as they are commonly known, are laid on the hair and hatch out quickly. The life cycle during the winter is only 10 days, so the numbers living in the horse's coat increase rapidly.

Treatment This consists of dusting the coat with any of the proprietary louse powders containing gamma benzine hexachloride or one of the newer organo-phosphorous compounds. This should be repeated in two weeks to kill the next generation of lice. Ivermectin is effective against lice.

Mange Mites

The only type of mange seen in horses in Great Britain is that due to a mite called *Chorioptes equi*. This mange mite infects the back of the fetlock area and is only seen in those horses with heavy feather. The mite lives in and on the skin causing scabbing and an intense itch, so horses who are affected spend their time stamping the ground in an attempt to get some relief.

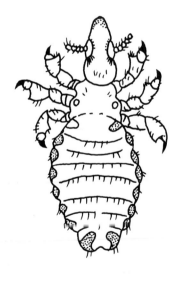
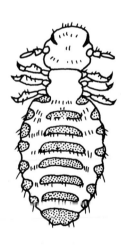

(a) (b)

Fig 57 Horse lice

(a) The sucking louse
(b) The biting louse

Treatment   Any organo-phosphorous based wash will give temporary alleviation, but a permanent cure is more difficult to achieve.

Harvest Mites

These small mites can cause an exudative (seeping) lesion on the pasterns of thin-skinned horses, especially young Thorough-breds. They develop during late summer, when the mites are at their most common and can be controlled by twice weekly treatments with an insecticidal wash.

Warbles

The Ministry of Agriculture, Fisheries and Food campaign to eradicate the warble fly from the cattle population of Great Britain has reduced the number of warble flies drastically and the condition is now rare in the horse. The warble fly lays its eggs on the horse's legs. Here they hatch out and burrow through the skin. Once under the skin they migrate up the legs to the back. As the horse is not the usual host of the warble fly, the larvae do not mature as they do in cattle, but form a hard lump, unfortunately nearly always under the saddle area. A poultice applied to the lump will sometimes encourage it to burst like an abscess, but often the only satisfactory treatment is surgical removal.

Nodular Skin Disease

Nodular skin disease is one of those skin conditions that does not belong in any group, but it is often confused with warble infestation. The condition is characterised by the sudden

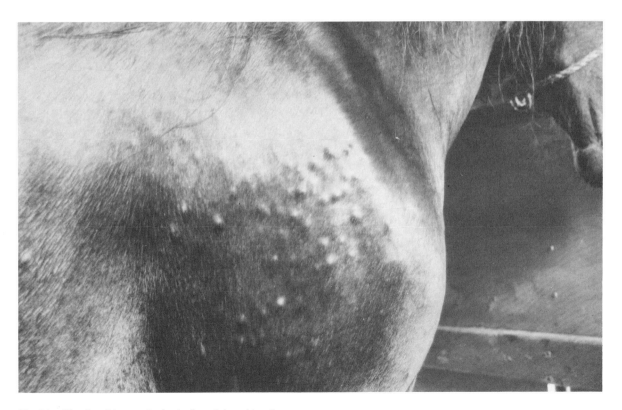

Fig 58   The hard lumps typical of nodular skin disease.

appearance of firm, painless nodules in the skin of the neck or back. The cause of this condition is not known, but microscopic examination of the lumps shows that the structured collagen (a fibrous protein) fibres of the skin become damaged and that the area is packed with cells normally associated with an allergic reaction.

Treatment   This involves removing the dead collagen. If this is carried out successfully, the lump gradually disappears. Sometimes this happens spontaneously and the dead collagen is pushed out as a plug; more rarely the condition disappears as quickly as it appeared, leaving the owner happy but the veterinary surgeon mystified as to the reason.

Aural Plaques

This skin condition is another oddity of which cause is unknown. The condition is seen in any breed and age of horse and affects the skin on the inside of the ear. White plaques of crusty material develop in collections. When this material is removed, a thickened pink skin is exposed. The lesions do not appear to be irritable, in that head shaking and ear twitching do not accompany them. In our experience, however, the lesions can occasionally be painful and the horse may resent any interference with the affected ear. The cause is thought to be a reaction to the bite of the small black flies that are found in the ear during the summer months. Once the plaques have developed, they remain indefinitely and no effective treatment has yet been found.

SKIN TUMOURS

Warts and Sarcoids

This group of tumours has long caused confusion amongst laymen and vets. When is a wart a wart and when is it a sarcoid?

Warts   Warts should be defined as the infectious disease cutaneous papillomatosis, which occurs in young horses. The warts (papillomata) appear on the nose and, less commonly, on other parts of the body, as small, hard, raised lumps, varying in number from a few to many hundred. The disease is caused by a virus which is specific to the horse. The precise method of infection is unknown, but it seems likely that the virus gains entry through insignificant skin abrasions. The young horse's habit of nuzzling various objects could result in small skin wounds which, in turn, could lead to infection and would then explain the high incidence of warts on the muzzle. The disease is self-limiting, and the warts, if left undisturbed, disappear 3 to 4 months after their first appearance.

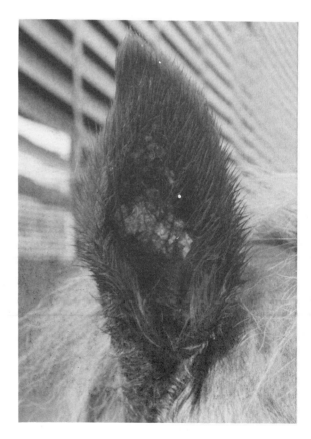

Fig 59   An aural plaque.

Sarcoids Sarcoids are not as easy to explain, either their cause or their make up. It is considered by some researchers that they are an exuberant growth of normal skin tissue, other researchers believe that sarcoids are neoplastic. The present view is that sarcoids are, in fact, locally invasive, non-spreading tumours of the skin. At first they look like a wart, but as they grow the skin covering the sarcoid becomes thin and breaks, allowing an ulcer to develop.

Sarcoids can occur anywhere on the body, either singly or at multiple sites and seldom undergo spontaneous remission. They are notoriously difficult to treat as they have a tendency to recur when removed by surgery. They should be treated with caution and it is unwise to consider purchasing a horse that has sarcoids.

The causal agent is again considered to be a virus but the interrelationship of virus and tumour is still not understood. It is possible that sarcoids develop as a result of earlier non-productive infection with the virus that causes juvenile warts or due to infection with the virus that causes warts in cattle. We know that after the inoculation of young horses with an extract of bovine papilloma virus, a sarcoid-like growth appears at that site.

Treatment Treatment of sarcoids is difficult. Where the site allows, surgical removal is the easiest method, but up to 50 per cent of sarcoids recur after surgical excision.

Cryosurgery is a better technique. The method generally used is to freeze the tumour with a liquid nitrogen spray or probe. The frozen tumour sloughs away and healing takes place over a period of three to eight weeks.

Radiation techniques have been developed at several specialised centres. Radioactive iridium pins or gold dust are implanted into the tumour mass and over the next 6 to 12 months the tumour gradually disappears. This method of treatment is especially valuable where surgery, either normal or cryo, cannot be

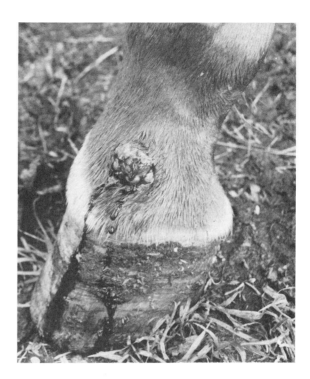

Fig 60   Cryosurgery will be needed to remove this sarcoid.

performed because of the position of the tumour. Tumours around the eye are an example.

Another method that has been developed to treat this type of sarcoid is the use of the human BCG vaccine. Normally used to vaccinate children against tuberculosis, it also has the property of stimulating local cell immunity. When it is injected into the base of a sarcoid the local reaction kills the tumour cells and the tumour starts to regress. Several treatments are needed before regression is complete and occasionally a severe reaction at the site of injection complicates the procedure.

Melanoma

This unpleasant tumour is found in the grey horse. It is a tumour of the melanin producing cells and can develop anywhere on the body, although the area under the tail and on the perineal area (between the anus and genital organs in the male, anus and udder in the female) and perianal regions are common sites.

Melanomas are frequently multiple and are first seen as small, firm, black lumps in the substance of the skin. They develop in three different ways. The most common pattern is a constant, slow growth over many years. The tumours remain local and do not metastasise (spread to other sites) but as they get larger the skin covering them becomes damaged and ulcers develop on the surface. The least common type is the tumour that is malignant from the start. This type quickly invades local tissue and spreads to nearby lymph nodes and from there to the lungs, liver and other organs. The third type of melanoma is that which has been quietly growing for many years and then suddenly becomes malignant and rapidly spreads through the body.

Surgery is the only method of treatment and this should not be undertaken lightly. The only type of tumour that is worth removing by surgery is the single tumour that shows no sign of malignancy and even these tend to have seeded before removal.

Squamous Cell Carcinoma

These tumours are malignant and appear on the surface of mucous membranes. They comprise the second largest group of tumours affecting horses and involve the eye and associated structures, the penis and sheath in males, and the vulva in females. The tumour spends a long time invading the local tissues before it spreads to other parts of the body. This allows effective surgical removal to be carried out.

ALLERGIC DISEASES

Contact Dermatitis

Every so often a horse can become sensitive to materials in direct contact with his skin. These agents can cause a direct dermatitis because of their caustic nature. The loss of hair from the soiled hind quarters of a scouring foal is a good example. More commonly, the skin becomes sensitive to the repeated presence of these agents. In these cases the more obvious symptoms of repeated exposure to the material are a dermatitis with inflammation, loss of hair, redness of the skin and a variable degree of self trauma.

The treatment consists of a thorough cleansing of the area with warm water and the removal of the offending substance from the environment of the horse. Which substance though? Synthetic materials are often to blame, common culprits are the dyes or preservatives in tack or blankets and fly sprays and medicaments. Many plant juices can also cause problems and the giant hog weed which grows along river banks is particularly toxic.

Sweet Itch

The disease is characterised by a localised dermatitis affecting the mane and poll and the root of the tail. In severe cases the shoulder area and hind quarters may be affected. Early in the development of the disease the skin becomes very thickened and filled with fluid and the intense irritation causes the horse to rub on any convenient post. At this stage a close look at the lesions will show many pustules with small blobs of serum oozing out on to the surface.

As the itch becomes worse and the rubbing constant, the hair is gradually lost and the skin develops a corrugated appearance, becoming ridged and scaly. The mane may be lost completely and the tail may consist of a few scraggy hairs.

All types and colours of horses are affected

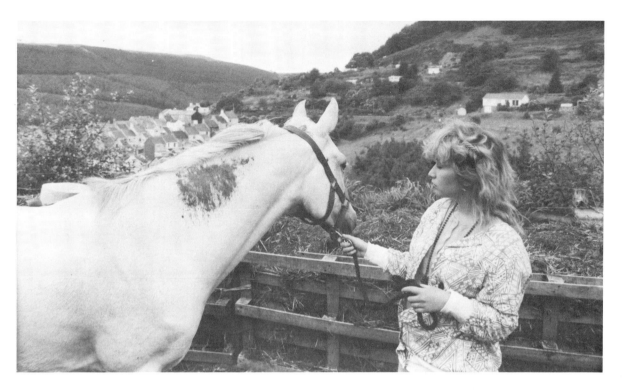

Fig 61　A case of contact dermatitis, probably caused by something the mare rubbed against.

but the pony and cob breeds seem to have a higher incidence. A family background of sweet itch is often present so it is possible that a hereditary factor is involved.

Once the condition has established itself it occurs each summer. The first lesions appear once the temperature starts to rise, only to regress again as the first frosts herald the start of winter. In the warmer south, the lesions reach two peaks of severity, one in June and again in September. Farther north the worst period seems to be July.

Causes　Many causes have been suggested, varying from an allergy, to grass proteins, to a reaction to microfilaria, worm larvae which live under the skin. Photosensitivity has also been incriminated.

The first clue to the probable cause of sweet itch is contained in some work published by Riek in 1972. He was investigating the cause of Queensland itch – a similar condition occurring in Australia – and demonstrated that it was due to an allergic reaction to the bite of the midge *Culicoides robertsi*.

Researchers in England then found that one midge called *Culicoides pulicaris* showed a preference for the upper body, a high proportion attacking the mane, withers and tail. This midge has a wide geographical distribution, its population peaks correspond to the periods of highest incidence of sweet itch and it feeds an hour before and after sunset. They concluded it was probably the culprit.

Treatment　Like most conditions that are difficult or impossible to cure, the list of possible treatments is endless. If the modern theory is correct, that the cause of sweet itch is an allergic reaction to the bites of the midge,

99

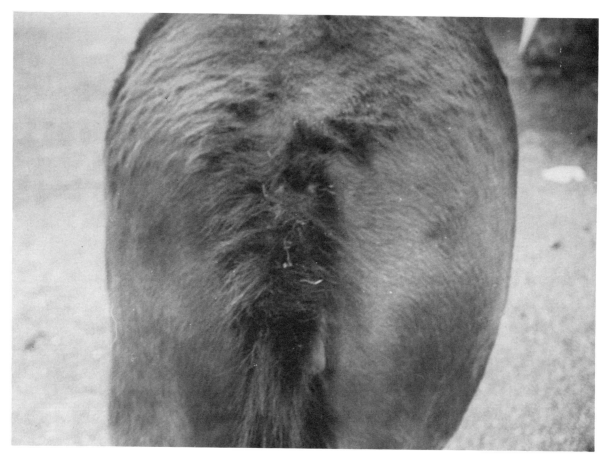

Fig 62   The scrubbed hair and scabby appearance of an early case of sweet itch.

treatment of the lesions is not likely to lead to a permanent cure. Each time the horse is exposed to a midge attack, a reaction starts and the lesions recur. However, a group of drugs can be used to control the inflammation and subsequent damage to the skin. Corticosteroid and antihistamine preparations are the most widely used. Their disadvantage is the frequency of application needed and their cost. Corticosteroid injections with a long-term action are the most useful for controlling the intense reactions present. Other lotions and remedies that are used are Benzyl Benzoate, Caladryl and Coal Tar lotions. Even sump oil has its advocates. All these treatments suffer from the same drawback, that their effect is temporary so daily application is necessary to ensure that they work.

The key to successful control of sweet itch is a simple one; the midge must be prevented from biting. Often, however, practical difficulties are involved. It has been demonstrated, time after time, that if the susceptible pony is stabled and midges are prevented from entering the stable by the use of screens and insecticide strips, sweet itch will not develop. However, how many people can afford to keep their pony in all summer? A partial solution is to stable the pony during the time of greatest risk, that is, in the early morning and

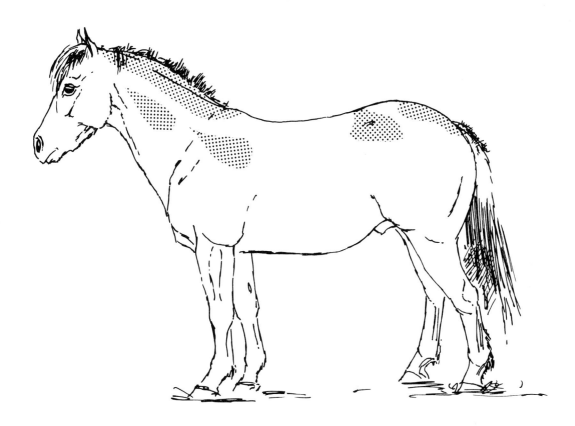

Fig 63 Areas usually affected by sweet itch (shaded).

from late afternoon until late evening, and to use one of the new synthetic pyrethrum insecticides to kill the midges before they feed. The best method is to spray the whole body surface of the pony with a solution of insecticide every two weeks, and every week during wet weather.

Various neck straps and head collar strips or tags, impregnated with insecticides, are available. They may work, but their effect may be too local to ensure that the sweet itch sufferer is never bitten.

The most exciting cure, and it will be a cure, is borrowed from human medicine. Great advances have been made in the human field in the blocking of the agents causing allergy. If we can identify the exact chemical that causes sweet itch it should be possible to produce blocking agents. Administered as a vaccine, these would prevent the allergen starting its allergic reaction.

Urticaria

This alarming condition is characterised by the sudden appearance of large weals on the skin. The muzzle, the ears, the vulva and sometimes the lower legs swell up. Very quickly the horse's condition looks distressing but in reality it is not serious. Treatment with an

101

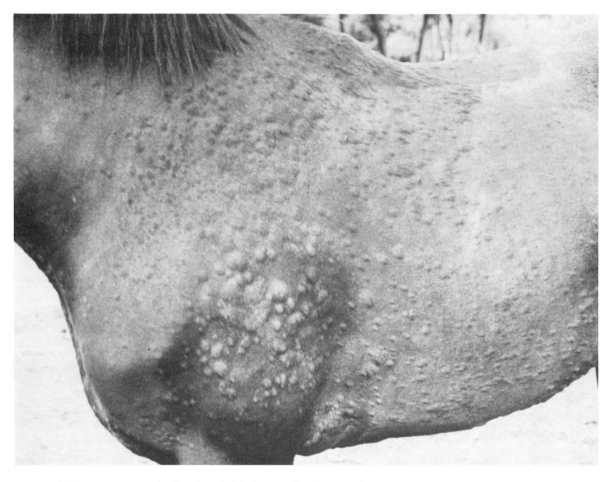

Fig 64   This severe case of urticaria subsided soon after treatment.

antihistamine preparation by injection will soon resolve the symptoms.

The condition is associated with a sudden change in the nature of the horse's food and often occurs shortly after spring turnout. The sudden intake of rich grass proteins upsets the system. A less severe condition follows inadvertent contact with young nettles. Presumably the horse does not notice the half-grown patch before starting to roll, thus collecting a few too many nettle stings. If the horse is obviously uncomfortable, showing signs of colic, sweating, breathing heavily and salivating, then do not wait but call for assistance at once. Urticaria can be one symptom of a systemic allergy to some foreign material, either a drug or some new food additive. Whatever the cause, the reaction is potentially serious and should be dealt with as soon as possible.

Photosensitivity

Photosensitivity, or the sensitisation of the skin to the ultra-violet rays of sunlight, is a condition caused by the presence of photo-active agents in the skin. These can gain entry in the feed, the weeds St John's Wort and Bog Asphodel are good examples, or they can build up in the system as a result of a malfunction of

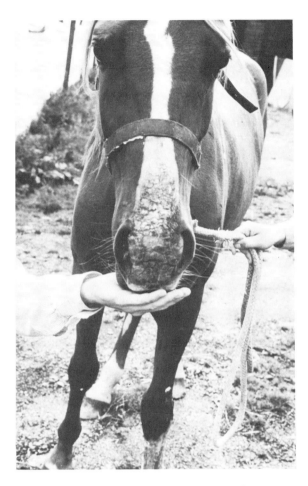

Fig 65   A severe case of photosensitivity. The left cannon is also affected.

the liver.

The chemicals react with the sunlight causing severe damage to the skin, especially those areas which are exposed to the direct rays of the sun. The muzzle, white feet and coronary band, the ears and any white areas are badly affected. The skin becomes swollen, hot and inflamed. Then, as it dies, it becomes hard and wrinkled and eventually will slough off.

Treatment   Systemic corticosteroids and antihistamines will, in the early stages, minimise the damage; local use of an antiseptic ointment will hasten the healing process. Immediate removal of the suffering horse to a darkened box is essential, to prevent further damage to the skin.

10 Locomotory System

LAMENESS

Causes

It is fashionable, when considering the causes of lameness in a forelimb, to talk of navicular disease and pedal osteitis; however, it is vital to remember that the vast majority of lamenesses result from infection in the foot. In addition, there are various conditions which are the result of trauma or physical damage to the solar surface of the foot. Bruising to the sole or bulbs of the heels can be caused by sudden impact on a rough surface where the horse is travelling too fast to tread carefully. It may also be a consequence of overreaching – when the forefoot is damaged by the hind foot as it lands. Where overreaching is severe, a wound may occur in the heel and a slice of heel may even be removed.

Another site of bruising is at the angle of the hoof, where the wall of the hoof at the heel doubles back to form the bar alongside the frog. A bruise in this area is commonly known as a corn, and often results from the pressure of an ill-fitting shoe. Bruising occurs at this point

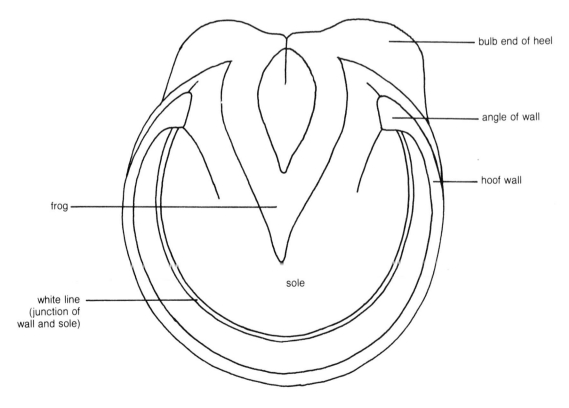

Fig 66   The normal foot

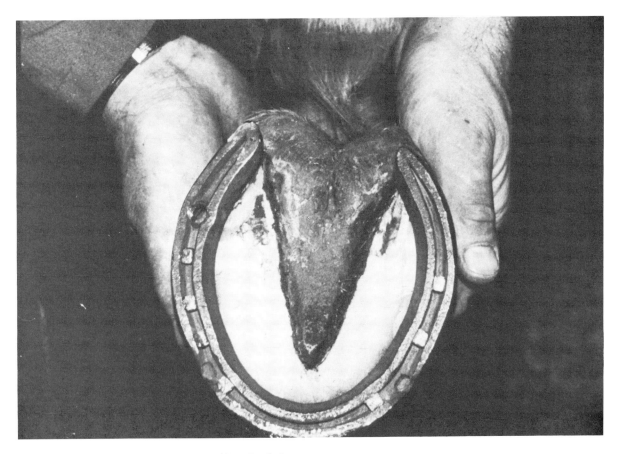

Fig 67   The well-shod foot with a good length of shoe.

because it corresponds with the heel of the shoe. If the shoe does not extend sufficiently far over the heel of the foot, it will put pressure on the angle. As the foot grows, the shoe obviously does not increase in size, so it is carried forward, being fixed at the toe. Consequently it becomes too short in relation to the foot. A shoe which is left on too long will therefore predispose the horse to corns. A shoe that has been made too short will have the same effect, and in this case a piece of stone or gravel under the shoe will cause a corn, as will a rough bearing surface rubbing on the foot.

Fast work on a hard surface by a horse with upright pasterns will have a concussive effect that may cause corns, recognised by a red discoloration of the horn tissue. Tissue damaged in such a way, no matter where it occurs in the foot, may subsequently become infected. Where the trauma is sufficiently severe, caused by a sharp stone or nail perhaps, the sole or frog may be penetrated and infection inevitably results. Usually there is a short period of acute lameness following the traumatic incident, after which the horse rapidly improves. However, usually four to five days later the lameness returns and becomes increasingly severe, sometimes with startling rapidity. A horse that has been completely sound in the morning may, by late afternoon, be virtually unable to put its foot to the ground. When the lameness is this severe, there are only two possible causes – either the horse has a broken bone, or he has pus in the foot.

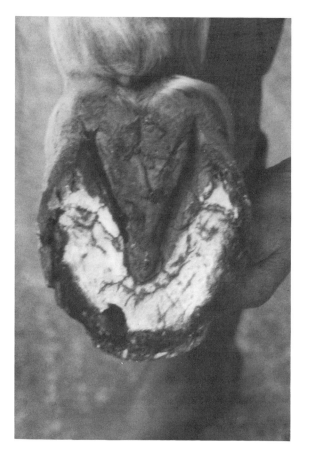

Fig 68 An infected sole requires good drainage.

pressure over the sole with hoof testers it is often possible to localise quite accurately the site of infection under the sole. It is always satisfying to release a jet of pus and, by creating adequate drainage, provide rapid relief, but often, where the infection is tracking slowly through the foot, the pus cannot be so easily drained.

By following a track from the solar surface of the hoof, the active site of infection can be located. Following such tracks in a sole that has hardened in a dry summer can be extremely difficult. In this situation 'tubbing', by standing the foot in warm water and magnesium sulphate, can be valuable in softening the hoof. Infections tracking up the leg, inside the hoof, break out of the leg at the first opportunity if left to develop by themselves. This opportunity arises at the coronary band, and when a point at the coronet softens and bursts, the site of penetration can frequently be found in the sole immediately below it.

On occasions the horse gives no clues as to the site of lameness. In this situation, shoulder lameness is a common diagnosis. It should be remembered that shoulder lamenesses are rare and when they do occur they are fairly obvious, even to the inexperienced observer.

Perhaps at this stage we should stop and consider how we go about identifying the site and cause of lameness that is not immediately obvious. It is as well to remember that to reach a final conclusion may be a lengthy procedure involving several hours on several days, so the whole process may take up to two weeks. On the whole, the more lame the horse, the quicker and easier it is to make a diagnosis. The difficult horses are the ones who are intermittently and unpredictably lame.

Where there has been no initial traumatic incident, the onset of lameness may be quite insidious. However, pus will form several days after the horse has been shod if a nail has been placed too close to the sensitive laminae, or when grit has started to track up the dead laminae following an episode of laminitis.

Diagnosis

Locating site While the horse, at this stage, will probably be showing obvious signs that the foot is the cause of his problems, occasionally he may not. There will usually be evidence of heat when the foot is felt, although this can sometimes be misleading. By applying

Recent history The more information the owner can give on the history of the lameness, the easier it is to reach a diagnosis. Such points as a recent fall or being cast in a box are obviously helpful, but even seemingly irrelevant points can be valuable. The horse's age may give a clue; splints, for example, do not occur in horses over seven years of age, for reasons which will become apparent later. Similarly joint infections, unless resulting from a penetrating wound, are predominantly a problem of foals. The type of work that a horse is doing will often give a clue. Sore shins are seen in the young Thoroughbred racing on a hard surface.

Stance and conformation It is valuable to stand back and look at the horse from a distance at an early stage. Much can be learned from the way he stands, whether he sits back on his hind legs with forelegs pushed out in front, as in laminitis, whether he shifts his weight from one leg to another, or whether the toe is pointed. At the same time, conformation may give some clues. Poor hock conformation predisposes to strains on the joint, which may result in curb or spavin formation. Short, upright pasterns can exacerbate concussion through the joints and arthritic conditions, while long, sloping pasterns increase the tension on the soft tissue structures behind the legs – the tendons and suspensory ligaments – increasing the likelihood of strains.

Movement The next stage is to look at the horse moving, probably first at the walk and then at the trot. This is done away from, towards and past the observer.

The first point is to identify on which leg the horse is lame. Even to the experienced eye, this is not always as easy as it would at first seem, particularly when the lameness involves more than one leg or arises from a back abnormality. By turning in a circle, first in one direction and then the other, the lameness may be exacerbated or decreased, depending on whether the lame leg is on the inside or outside of the circle. By tightening the circle this can become more pronounced. Where a hind limb lameness is present, however, the results are not nearly as conclusive. Much can be gained from noting whether the leg is moved through an arc

(abducted) away from the body and whether all the phases of stride are shortened. Also examine how the foot hits the ground: where the heel area is involved, the toe will come down first and vice versa.

Comparison Next, compare the features of each leg closely with those of the opposite leg, first visually and then by manipulation. Often the problem will be seen to occur where differences arise.

First consider the feet. They should be a pair, when similarly trimmed or dressed and, looked at from the side, should have a similar length of heel and hoof/pastern axis (that is, the line from fetlock through the coronet and down the front of the hoof should be straight). Where one foot is large and the other contracted, the problem will nearly always lie in the contracted hoof. This is because the extra growth in the heel area is a result of less weight being applied through the chronically lame foot. The frog does not then come into contact with the ground surface, so that pressure is not applied to the underlying digital cushion in walking and the walls of the heel are therefore not expanded to the normal extent.

Turn the foot up and look at the shoes. Uneven wearing indicates that the foot is not being placed squarely.

Other techniques By this stage, the cause of lameness has usually become apparent, but on occasions further techniques may need to be employed for a correct diagnosis. The site of the pain can be identified by injecting local anaesthetic around the nerves at specific sites as they run down the leg. By blocking the nerve, sensation at any point further down the leg supplied by that nerve is lost. Nerves are blocked in sequence up the leg, but each block is a time-consuming procedure, so more than one visit is sometimes necessary. Local anaesthetic can also be injected into a joint or around a suspected bony swelling to see whether this eliminates the pain.

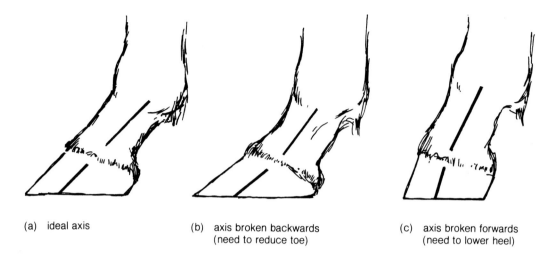

(a) ideal axis

(b) axis broken backwards
     (need to reduce toe)

(c) axis broken forwards
     (need to lower heel)

Fig 69   The hoof/pastern axis of a riding horse.

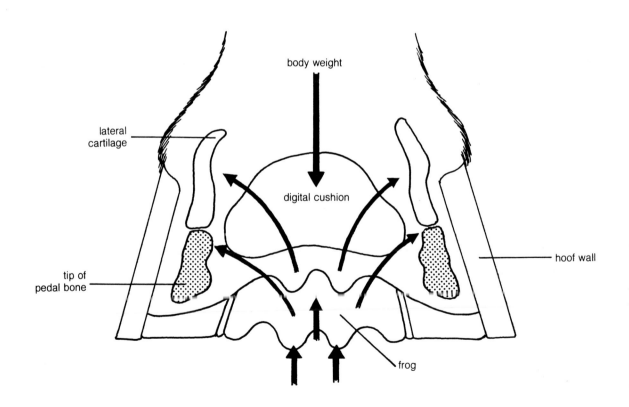

Fig 70   Section through the foot demonstrating the function of the central digital cushion.

By locating the general site of lameness we can then have a fair idea of where to direct our X-ray machine. X-rays enable us to look inside the leg, particularly at the bony structures, but to a lesser extent at the surrounding tissues. Usually by this stage a final conclusion has been reached, but even more sophisticated diagnostic techniques may now be employed. Although bone appears dense and inactive, this is far from the truth. Where there is damage to bone, regenerative activity is increased within the bony structure. It is now possible to inject into the blood a radioactive marker attached to a carrier which is selectively taken up by bone. Damaged, and therefore more active bone will take up more marker. Consequently by running a scintillation counter over the bones, to measure the radiation, high levels of activity can be accurately pinpointed, demonstrating the site of injury.

FORELIMB LAMENESS

Returning to specific conditions of the foreleg which are commonly encountered and cause lameness, it is logical to start at the foot and work up the leg.

Thrush

Thrush is a malodorous, degenerative condition of one or more frogs, in horses kept under conditions of poor management on dirty, damp bedding. Poor trimming of the hoof further exacerbates the condition. An unpleasant black discharge issues from the grooves in the frog and indicates infection by several types of bacteria. Only in the more severe cases is lameness present. Proper cleaning of the foot on a daily basis, together with clean bedding, results in rapid recovery.

Sand Cracks

Sand cracks, grass cracks or quarter cracks are cracks in the wall of the hoof which start at the ground, on the bearing surface of the hoof wall, and extend, to a varying extent, up the hoof. Where the crack extends on to the coronary band, a serious problem exists. The crack is caused by neglected feet in which insufficient trimming has resulted in a splitting of the wall at ground level. Thin or excessively dry hooves are at greater risk. The crack is obvious and may or may not cause lameness. It is easy for the underlying tissue to become infected.

Treatment   Various methods of treatment are employed. Where the crack does not extend up the full length of the hoof, a hot iron placed horizontally across the top of the crack may prevent further spread but success is limited. Quarter clips applied on each side of the crack help to keep the walls rigid. By trimming the hoof back in the area of the crack, pressure is taken off the crack, so that further expansion is reduced. Where these lines of treatment have not been successful, the movement between the two sides of the crack can be halted. The crack is reamed out and a line of holes drilled down each side of the crack. Wire or tape is used to lace the crack which is filled with epoxy glue. The whole lot is then allowed to grow out, a procedure which may take 6–12 months. However, provided that the coronet is not split, there is a good chance of full eventual recovery.

Laminitis

Laminitis is a condition which usually affects two or more feet, and frequently the forefeet are involved most severely. Nevertheless, the hind feet *can* be primarily involved and occasionally only one foot may be damaged.

Traditionally, laminitis is a condition of the fat pony with a large crest, grazing lush grass

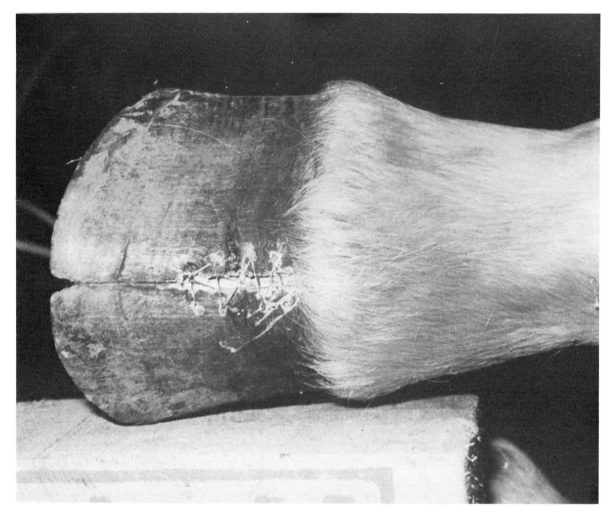

Fig 71   A sandcrack, repaired by lacing with wire before gluing with acrylic.

in spring or autumn. However, much change of thought has recently occurred regarding all aspects of this condition.

Laminitis can be defined as damage to the laminae of the hoof. The laminae are the interlocking leaves of tissue that attach the hoof wall to the underlying pedal bone. It used to be considered that laminitis was the result of inflammation of the laminae. However, recent studies have demonstrated that a short period of inflammation is followed by congestion, or stagnation, of blood in the laminae. As a result,

the blood supply short-circuits the hoof at the coronet and the hoof is deprived of nutrients and oxygen; the living laminar tissue then dies. At this stage the hoof wall will not be hot, and the heat will be confined to the coronet.

Why is the intake of grass in fat ponies, in the spring and autumn, reflected in these changes in the feet? An excess of carbohydrate intake, as occurs in the ingestion of rapidly growing spring (or more commonly, autumn) grass, is only one of a variety of causes. These causes also include excessive corn intake, infection

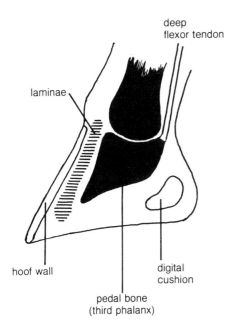

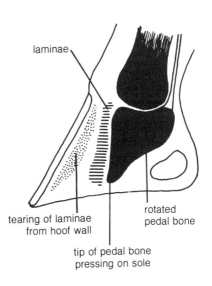

Fig 72   Section through hoof, showing pedal bone and laminae in a healthy state.

Fig 73   Section through hoof, showing damage caused by laminitis.

resulting from failure to lose all the foetal membranes after foaling, or intestinal infections. Fatty liver syndrome – a condition of obese ponies – is also a cause, since the liver is important in detoxifying the blood. When carbohydrates are fed, lactate is produced in excess in the gut. This increases the acidity of the gut. The normal bacteria involved in digestion are killed. As they break up, these bacteria produce poisons (endotoxins); endotoxins affect the blood flow rate, which is most obviously manifested at the extremities – namely the feet. Similar poisons are released during a septicaemic infection, where the toxins invade the blood system. In cases where only one foot is involved, laminitis usually follows a blow to the outside of the hoof wall, causing bruising within the underlying laminae.

In the acute stages of the disease signs are fairly non-specific. The pony shows unwillingness to eat, is markedly depressed and often does not want to stand. To take pressure off the painful forefeet, a characteristic stance is adopted, in which the weight is taken on the hind quarters and the forelegs are pushed out in front, so that all the weight is on the heels. As a result, with time, the toe grows much longer than the heels. Often the pony may be sweating and breathing hard and the condition may be confused with colic. The depression may cause a state similar to that produced by liver failure, further confused by the fact that the two conditions often occur together.

If the blood supply to the laminae is reduced, the new horn being formed is faulty and this can be demonstrated later by circumferential rings around the hoof wall known as 'laminitic rings'. As the horn grows, the debris accumulated in the damaged laminae separates the horn from the underlying pedal bone, so that the bone rotates around its point of attachment, the coffin joint, and its tip is pushed against the sole of the foot, applying pressure on the sole from above. The normally concave sole is thus flattened. If this process is allowed to continue, the pedal bone may penetrate the sole and the future outlook is very bleak. The

111

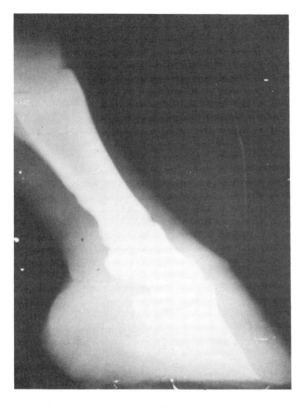

Fig 74   X-ray showing the tilting of the tip of the pedal bone which applies pressure to the sole.

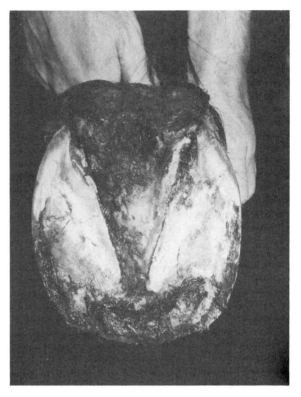

Fig 75   Penetration of the sole by a rotated pedal bone.

degree of the pedal bone's rotation is therefore an important indication of the likely outcome.

Treatment   The long-term changes start to occur within four hours of onset of the disease, so rapid treatment is essential. Treatment is based on several principles:

1   Removal of the causal factor. If this includes excessive eating, a purgative may be required, together with a much reduced diet. Complete starvation will, however, result in a sudden fat release in the liver and subsequent liver failure, which only makes the condition worse.

2.   Relief of pain. The condition is very painful due to the lack of blood supply to the hoof. It is similar to the acute pain experienced when very cold fingers are placed in hot water.

3.   Re-establishment of the blood supply to the hoof. This is best done by making the horse walk on a flat, not too soft surface. The pressure on the frog and underlying digital cushion act as a pump, pushing blood round the foot. The old practice of standing the foot in cold water should not be followed as this will reduce the blood supply. If anything, warming the foot would be better.

4.   Prevention of rotation of the pedal bone by stopping the toe from becoming overlong and lowering the heels. It may be beneficial to use a heart bar shoe. This is an ordinary shoe with a heart-shaped bar under the frog which supports the pedal bone over it. In the long term, the original shape of the foot will not be

112

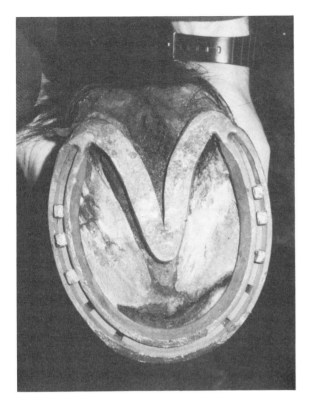

Fig 76   The heart bar shoe supports the pedal bone during laminitis.

completely restored until all the debris in the laminae is removed. This can only be done by the drastic step of stripping off the hoof wall in sections, back to the living tissue, and allowing new horn to grow straight down. Following recovery there is a strong tendency to recurrence, and strict attention must be paid to diet, exercise and foot care. Dietary supplementation with methionine, to improve growth of healthy horn, is also valuable.

Pedal Bone Fracture

Fracture of the pedal bone occurs more commonly in the forefoot than the hind. It usually results from a blow, particularly if combined with a twisting action as the foot lands. This may happen when landing on a sharp, pointed

stone, for example. The significance of the injury depends primarily on whether or not the coffin joint is involved. Where it *is* involved, the situation is much more serious. The problem is that the bone is completely encased in hoof, so diagnosis can only be confirmed by X-ray examination. The hoof also makes treatment very difficult, since although it is semi-rigid it will not immobilise the fracture sufficiently and access to the bone is hampered. Nevertheless, the pedal bone can be screwed across the fracture if necessary, but this should be done at an early stage. It is usually adequate, however, to render the hoof completely rigid by applying a surgical shoe with a bar across the back and quarter clips which prevent the hoof from expanding when weight is applied.

Navicular Disease

Navicular disease is a condition generally regarded with great fear as being progressive and untreatable. It is a too frequently diagnosed, chronic lameness, usually involving both forelimbs. The disease results from damage to the blood supply to the navicular bone. This damage takes the form of thrombosis or blockage of the blood vessels. As a result, food supply to the bone is compromised and the bone degenerates. Degeneration is painful and results in lameness. An alternative blood supply is often established but not at the same rate as destruction occurs. Small holes or channels appear in the bone and can be seen on X-ray, not to be confused with nutrient channels in the bone.

The condition usually appears during the maximum working period, particularly where the work is at irregular intervals. Lameness is insidious in onset, but it often improves as work progresses. With time, however, the interval before the improvement starts, is increased. Sometimes the lameness is acute in onset and affects one foot in particular, starting during cantering.

Diagnosis Diagnosis is difficult but relies on specific changes being demonstrated by X-ray in the navicular bones. It must be stressed, however, that these changes occur in horses showing no sign of lameness, in which case the horse is not considered to have navicular disease; nor will the disease inevitably follow.

The lameness can be localised to the area of the navicular bone by blocking the nerves to that area using local anaesthesia. Often at this point the horse appears to be lame on the other leg, and indeed he is, since the horse was originally lame on both forelegs but lameness becomes evident in the less severely affected leg only when the pain in the more severely affected one is blocked.

The changes described result from excessive strain placed on the soft tissue attachments (ligaments) to the navicular bone by repeated over-extensions of the joint. Where the heels have been allowed to become low and weak, and the toe long, blood flow is considerably slowed. This state results from shoes not being fitted long enough at the heels or being left on too long before the foot is trimmed. When the navicular bone becomes painful, the horse raises its heel to reduce the tension. The horn therefore grows longer and the foot becomes contracted so that when weight is applied, the foot does not expand properly and blood flow is not adequately re-established.

Treatment It is necessary to correct the shoeing by providing plenty of length over the heels and by using a wide shoe to allow expansion. In the upright, boxy foot it may be necessary to cut vertical grooves down the hoof wall to allow expansion. Sometimes it is valuable to join the heels of the shoe behind the frog, providing extra support without applying frog pressure – an egg bar shoe.

The re-establishment of the blood supply medically is also helpful. Warfarin acts by dissolving clots and, used in carefully monitored doses, can be very helpful. The main drawbacks are that treatment must be constantly monitored and given daily over an indefinite period. Warfarin is also a prohibited substance in competitions.

Alternatively, the blood vessels to the area can be dilated using Isoxsuprine. This drug, given in a paste by mouth over six to fourteen weeks, is frequently permanently, or semi-permanently, effective in suppressing lameness. However, it is expensive.

An outdated method of treatment is to cut the posterior digital nerves to the area (popularly known as de-nerving) so that although the condition still exists, no pain is experienced. This is not recommended since the horse, losing sensation in part of his foot, is more likely to stumble.

Most recently, limited success has been achieved by surgically cutting the two ligaments that support the sides of the navicular bone. As a result, the tension on the bone is relaxed and the blood vessels supplying it, being less stretched, are presumably better able to service the bone.

Where chronic changes have occurred involving the surrounding structures none of these forms of treatment is likely to be completely successful. The important point to remember is that with proper foot care, the condition is preventable.

Pedal Osteitis

Pedal osteitis is another foot condition causing lameness. There is some debate over whether the condition actually exists. It is normally regarded as a thinning and irregularity of the toe region of the pedal bone, due to inflammation, and there may also be roughening of the ground surface of the bone in the heel area; this may result from infection or concussion. Infection often follows recurrent or deep corns in the sole overlying this area. The bone becomes concussed and bruised and new bone forms. Concussion is more likely where there are upright heels so that frog pressure is reduced, as is the hydraulic action of the blood in the foot overlying it. Puncture wounds may also cause concussion. The significance of new bone formation is the point in debate.

Treatment This is not very successful. Shoeing using protective pads must be the most helpful and a bar, applying pressure across the frog, is valuable to improve circulation. The drawbacks to cutting the nerve supply to the area, as a form of treatment, have already been described.

Fractures

Fractures of the pedal bone have already been discussed. Due to its strong square shape, fractures of the second phalanx are rare in horses in Great Britain. In the United States, where working horses are frequently turning sharply in barrel racing and cutting, the fracture is much more common. The pastern bone or first phalanx is more likely to fracture in horses in Britain, reflecting the waisted shape of the bone.

Where a single spiral split is present, it can be repaired by screwing across the split. This is less successful where a joint surface is involved in the split. Sometimes the bone will shatter into a mass of small pieces resembling a bag of marbles. Attempts to repair this type of injury are hopeless. All these injuries cause an acute lameness which is very sudden in onset, often during work.

It is becoming increasingly common to try to repair fractures of the metacarpal or metatarsal (cannon) bone, where the fracture is simple and the joints at the ends are not involved. This is usually done by screwing across the fracture line and may involve using metal plates applied along the length of the bone and screwed to support the bone. Sometimes it is surprisingly difficult to locate a crack in the bone and numerous X-rays may need to be taken at slightly varying angles to pick up a crack. Incomplete cracks in the bone surface may result from the stress of concussion when

a young horse whose bone structure is less dense is galloped on a hard surface. Most stress will occur when the horse lands on its forelegs and the weight is transmitted down the front of the cannon bone, creating a reaction, with heat and swelling down the front of the bone and acute pain. This condition, commonly known as sore shins, forces a relatively high proportion of young Thoroughbreds to end their first season's flat racing prematurely.

Splints

Running down each side of the top two-thirds of the cannon bone, slightly towards the back, are two narrow bones, the vestiges of the second and fourth digits of the evolving horse. They are attached to the cannon bone in early life by a fibrous ligament as the splint bones. If the horse is worked hard on a firm surface, the knee bones, which overlap the top of the splint bone, may put extra pressure on the splint bone causing the ligament to tear. Localised bleeding will occur which will form first a soft swelling, then a bony swelling or splint, which will fine down over a period of months. Although during splint formation there may be a period of lameness, lameness is rare once the swelling is formed, unless the new bone interferes with overlying structures. Between five and seven years of age the ligament becomes bony, so that tearing cannot occur. Consequently, splints cannot be formed after this has happened.

It has been suggested that where there is a dietary calcium deficiency, calcium may be removed from the outer layers of the bone, causing a loosening of the ligament, and that this may then predispose the ligament to tearing. It is important to differentiate splints from the normal, small, bony 'button' in which the splint bone frequently ends.

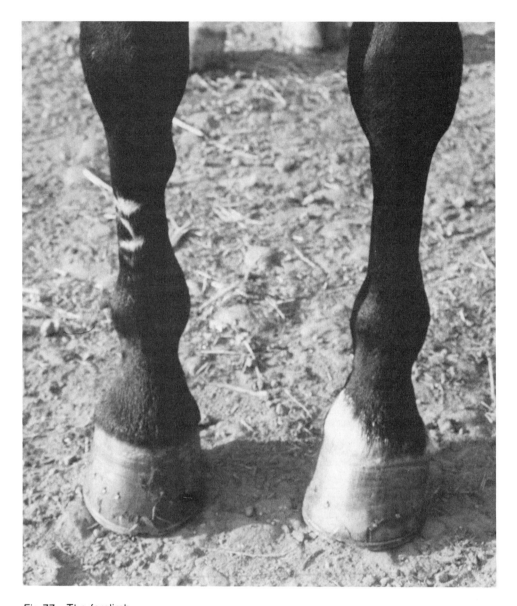

Fig 77   The forelimb

Big Leg

At this point we will consider the causes of a 'big leg'. This term is used to describe a thickening of the leg between the knee and fetlock or, less commonly, hock and fetlock. Such a reaction is usually accompanied by severe lameness.

It is important to remember that bone damage will cause this reaction, but the most common cause is a local reaction to infection in the foot which is spreading up the leg. This is particularly likely to be the cause where the pastern area is also swollen. Mud fever is a skin infection which can cause massive swelling and acute lameness.

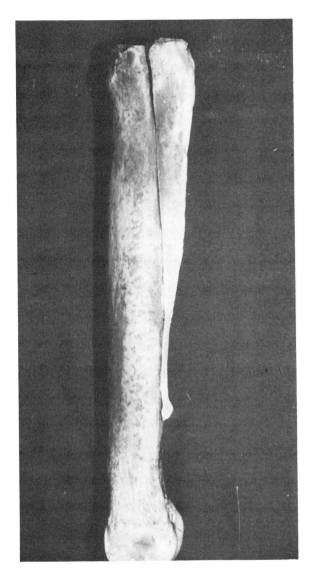

Fig 78   A side view of the cannon and splint bones. Note the normal button at the end of the splint bone.

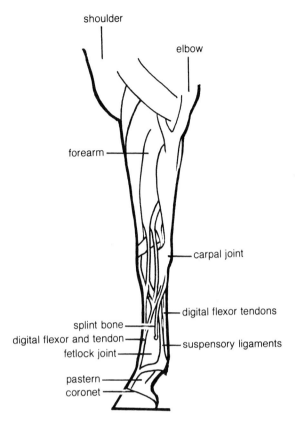

Fig 79   Structure of the lower forelimb.

Tendon Strain

The cause of lameness most often considered first is damage to the tendons, suspensory ligaments or both, running down the back of the leg. Tendons are composed of a mass of tiny fibrils running in sheaths longitudinally down the back of the leg from the muscles above the knee, to become attached to the bone at the foot. They have limited elastic properties; they can stretch over a very short period of time, as the weight of the horse moving through the air is brought to a standstill when the foot hits the ground. In so doing, they prevent the joints from extending too far and act as shock absorbers.

The muscle at the top of the tendon also tenses before landing and helps to absorb some of the energy. However, when the muscles are tired, they fail to absorb so much energy. If the ground surface is very hard, the foot cannot sink so far into it, and more strain is placed on the tendon. In these circumstances, some of the fibrils may rupture. The number that ruptures may vary from a very few, showing only a slight swelling and heat around the tendon sheath, to complete separation of the two ends of the tendon.

Treatment Whatever the injury, treatment is aimed at reducing the inflammation to a minimum in the early stages. This is done by reducing the blood supply to the area with cold applications, by using anti-inflammatory drugs and by prolonged periods of rest. Attempts to speed up healing in the later stages, either by firing or by splitting the tendons, have been demonstrated in ponies to be either of no benefit, or positively harmful, causing further unnecessary pain. Because the blood supply to tendons is very poor, recovery from these injuries can, in the most severe cases, take years to be complete. The recent use of carbon fibre, implanted into the tendon to provide a framework around which new tendon can form, has proved beneficial in some cases.

Since most (60 per cent) of the horse's weight is taken on the forelegs, tendon injuries usually occur in the forelegs. Damage to the suspensory ligaments which run initially to the sesamoid bones at the back of the fetlock, is similar in nature. In this case however, the support to the fetlock may be lost and the fetlock sinks close to the ground.

Such injuries can also arise from the horse overreaching and striking into the back of the forelegs with the hind legs during galloping.

Where the suspensory ligament attaches to the top of the sesamoid bones behind the fetlock, the sesamoid may be put under great strain. The ligament may tear off the top of the sesamoid or even cause the sesamoid to split so that the ligament takes a piece of bone with it. Such sesamoiditis carries a poor prospect of complete recovery.

Windgalls

Soft swellings may occur in a similar site at the back of the top of the fetlock joint but without causing lameness. These 'windgalls' or 'wind puffs' are swellings of the joint or sheath around the tendon. They are evident in many hard-working horses. They disappear during work and reappear after a period of rest. Occasionally they may result from dietary deficiencies, but in most cases they are caused by mild increases in work. Attempts to drain windgalls are usually unsuccessful and apart from being unsightly they are not usually significant. Another common site of windgalls is over the hock.

Ringbone

In the same way that the suspensory ligament can tear off the sesamoid bones under tension, so the tendons and ligaments may tear from their points of attachment on the first and second phalanges. Bleeding occurs at the site of tearing and eventually a bony mass occurs at the site. Old, deep wire cuts may produce a similar response.

Where these bony enlargements do not cross a joint, they are called false ringbones, high or low depending on whether they are present on the first or second phalanges. True ringbones cross the corresponding joint spaces, 'high' involving the pastern and 'low' the coffin joints. Six weeks will elapse before the tearing results in new bone being laid down. Once the swelling has reduced, most cases will recover unless the new bone involves vital structures overlying it.

The extent of the bony enlargement can be fully demonstrated only by using X-rays. Where a joint is involved, the situation is more serious, since the pain of moving the joint may render the horse chronically lame.

Broken Knee

Passing further up the foreleg, abnormalities become progressively less common. Injuries to the knee, however, are quite frequent and easily seen. 'Broken knee' is caused by lacerations or tears in the skin over the front of the knee, from a fall on a hard surface – usually the road. Often a bald area of scar tissue remains permanently at the site. This can only be removed by cosmetic surgery.

Where the knee is banged on the front, for example during a jump, there may be fluid enlargement of the joint or tendon sheaths running over the knee. Usually these will reduce with rest but there may be a permanently unsightly blemish left, even without lameness. Such swellings are generally known as carpitis.

In severe traumatic incidents, chips may be fractured from one or more of the bones of the knee. Initially the horse is acutely lame, but the lameness often resolves with rest, only to recur when work is resumed. These fractures usually need to be diagnosed by X-ray and the chips either removed or screwed back into place. Any subsequent arthritic changes will restrict movement in the joint.

Angular Leg Deformities

The legs of young foals, and occasionally of older horses, may appear bent when viewed from the front. The 'bend' often appears to originate at the knees and may affect one or both legs. The actual change in direction occurs at the growth plate of the radius immediately above (proximal to) the knee. The majority of such deviations of the lower leg bones are outwards (carpal valgus), giving a knock-kneed appearance, but occasionally they may be inwards (carpal varus), producing bandy legs.

Deformities that develop in older foals may follow traumatic injury to one leg; alternatively, prolonged, excessive weight may have been applied to one leg, where chronic lameness in the opposite leg has caused the animal to keep weight off it. A diet which causes too rapid growth can also be responsible for deviations of both limbs. Similar deviations can be seen in the hock and fetlock joints.

Angular limb deformities are most frequently seen at birth and the majority correct themselves. While it is important to allow time for spontaneous correction, it is essential to ensure that the situation is carefully monitored; appropriate corrective action can be taken where necessary to prevent the leg from being left permanently bent. Initially, conservative measures such as the application of splints or casts can be taken, together with frequent corrective hoof rasping. Where these are unsuccessful, recourse to surgery will be necessary.

Since the deviation results from excessive growth of one side of the growth plate, surgical treatment is based on preventing further growth on the faster growing side, or stimulating growth on the slower growing side. Growth is prevented by placing metal staples across the growth plate. A more successful variation is to place a screw on each side of the growth plate, with a figure of eight wire between. A third and simpler technique is to cut the periosteum, the layer of skin-like tissue on the surface of the bone, on the inside of the 'bend', which stimulates further growth on that side. Obviously any surgery must be completed well before bone growth has ceased, and early consultation with your vet is advised on this matter.

SHOULDER LAMENESS

Despite a general opinion to the contrary, shoulder lameness is extremely rare. In most cases, it is very obvious that the shoulder is the site of lameness, either because there is acute and painful swelling in that area, or because damage to the nerve supply to the area has caused the shoulder to drop or the surrounding muscle to waste away. If there is no obvious sign of lameness in the shoulder, you would be well advised to search elsewhere for the cause of the lameness.

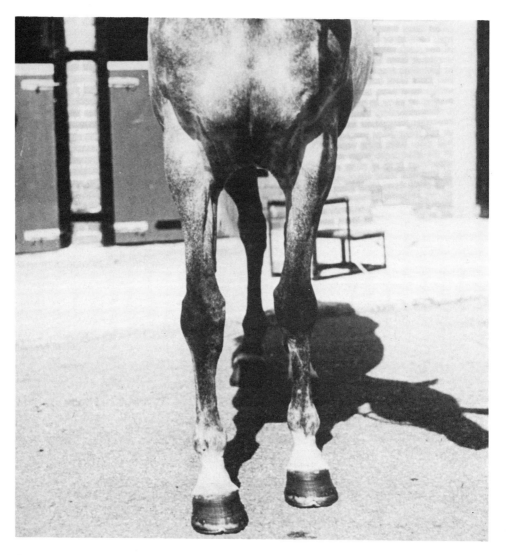

Fig 80   Angular deviation of the leg, originating at the knee. This requires correction before bone growth has ceased.

HIND LIMB LAMENESS

Fortunately, lameness in the hind limbs is much less common than in the forelimbs, but diagnosis of lameness is very much more difficult. Often both hind limbs are affected, so that neither leg is obviously producing lameness. Other signs may even suggest that the problem is in the back.

Although infection in the foot is again the most common cause of lameness in the hind limb, other foot problems are less common. This is probably because only forty per cent of the horse's weight is supported by the hind limbs. The hind limbs provide the power which propels the horse forward, using the massive muscles over the hind quarters. As a result, it is this area which is frequently the site of lameness.

is more common in horses with sickle or cow hocks. The lower two joints of the hock are usually affected. The condition is characterised by a bony swelling low down on the inside of the hock. The swelling can be of variable size and may not even be visible. If this is the case, there is only a characteristic opening of the joint spaces visible on X-ray. Once the new bone has formed and the joint becomes fused, the horse will become sound (although he may move with a slightly stiffened action), since it is the movement in the degenerating joint which is painful. Treatment is therefore based on speeding this renewing and fusing process as much as possible. Where practical, increased work can be used to speed

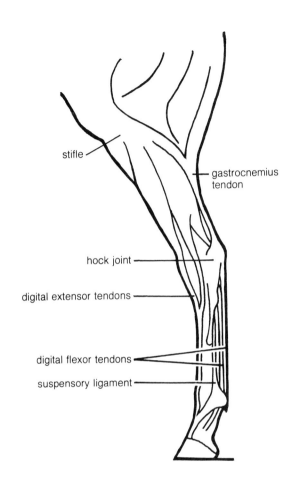

Fig 81 The hind limb

stifle

gastrocnemius tendon

hock joint

digital extensor tendons

digital flexor tendons

suspensory ligament

Hock Lameness

The hock is a common site of lameness. This is probably because the weight is not passed straight down through the joint – mechanical forces change direction markedly so that abnormal strains can easily occur at this point.

Bone spavin Bone spavin is one condition arising from such strains. Although trauma to the joint can cause a similar result, bone spavin

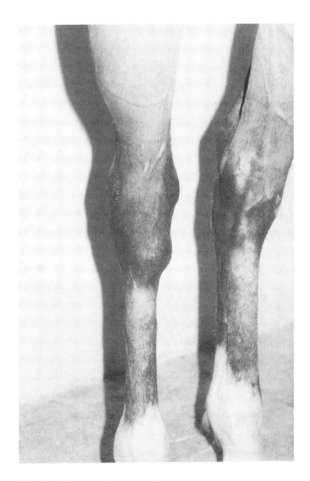

Fig 82 Severe bone spavin

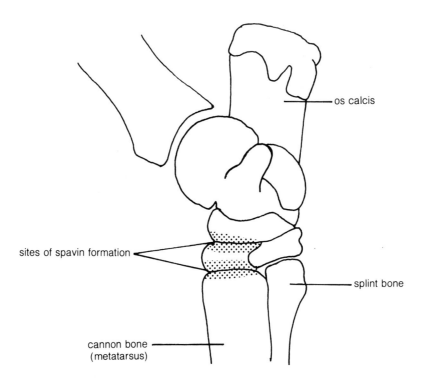

os calcis

sites of spavin formation

splint bone

cannon bone
(metatarsus)

Fig 83 Topographical anatomy of the hock.

the process, but if the horse is too lame, surgical intervention to drill out the joint surfaces causes a more rapid degenerative change and fusion occurs more quickly.

Bog spavin Bog spavin is a chronic enlargement of parts of the joint capsule of the hock, causing a soft swelling high on the outside, and low on the inside, of the joint. Occasionally a third swelling is present on the inside of the joint. The cause may be poor conformation, with the joint being too upright, a traumatic injury or a mineral imbalance, particularly of calcium and phosphorus, in the diet. usually the condition does not cause lameness unless bone damage has occurred during trauma. Treatment is often unsuccessful, particularly where the cause is poor conformation. Where this condition arises in young horses, it often resolves spontaneously.

Attention should be paid to correct mineral supplementation in the diet.

Curbs Curbs also arise from traumatic injury or poor conformation. A curb is an enlargement of the plantar ligament which runs down the back of the hock joint, directly below the point of the hock. The enlargement is just below the level of the hock joint. Sickle or cow-shaped hocks place abnormal strains on the ligament, predisposing the horse to curbs. Again, curbs are particularly common in young horses and often resolve spontaneously.

Lameness is usually restricted to the early, acute stage and is usually absent in the latter stages, even when the enlargement is quite marked. The importance of curbs is probably exaggerated. Treatment in the early stages is aimed at reducing inflammation, but in the

122

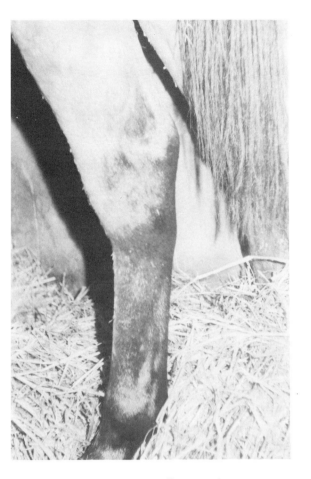

Fig 84 A curb does not usually cause lameness once the initial inflammation has subsided.

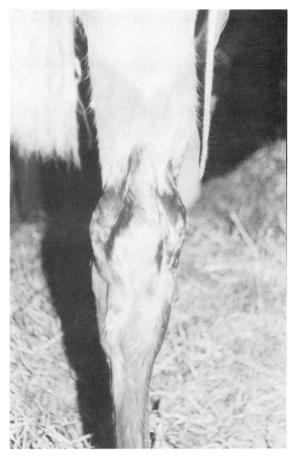

Fig 85 Very large thoroughpins can be frustratingly difficult to remove successfully.

chronic stage treatment is usually unnecessary and unrewarding.

Thoroughpin Where a soft fluid swelling of variable size is present in the angle of the hock, to either side and in front of the Achilles tendon, it is called a thoroughpin. This is caused by an enlargement of the flexor tendon sheath. When the hock is flexed, the bog spavin will reduce in size as the joint opens, but the thoroughpin will increase as space round the tendon is restricted. Usually only one hock is affected, the condition resulting from a blow. It is unlikely to cause lameness unless bone

damage has been done at the same time. Once again these swellings can be very difficult to reduce. If both hocks are affected, this probably means that the hocks are too upright. Where the horse is chronically lame, the chances of recovery are poor.

Capped hock Swelling at the point of the hock is the result of trauma at this point and is known as capped hock. The trauma usually arises from rubbing on a wall or trailer gate or from kicking back. Lameness is not usually a feature of this condition but the thickening of the skin over the area and the underlying fluid

123

swelling are usually permanent. To be successful, treatment must be started early, but it is advisable to avoid surgery as a wound breakdown, very likely at this site, will leave a blemish that is worse than the original.

Stifle lameness Lameness in the stifle is uncommon and difficult to diagnose. One condition, however, is not infrequently seen. This is an upward fixation of the patella; that is, a locking of the kneecap. To understand this, some knowledge of the stay apparatus is required.

The stay apparatus is a series of ligaments which join the bones of the hind limb in such a way that when one joint is moved, all the joints of the limb move with it and, more important, when one joint is fixed, all are fixed. This is very important since if one joint can be locked without using any muscle tension, the whole leg is fixed and the horse can relax completely and sleep in the standing position. This is achieved by hooking the inner condyle or knob of the thigh bone (femur) under a loop; the loop is formed by two of the three ligaments which connect the lower edge of the patella to the top of the tibia (the bone which connects the hock to the stifle). When weight is applied to the femur, the loop is pulled taut and the patella cannot slip off. To release this lock, the horse must first lift his weight off the femur, then contract the muscle running to the top of the patella, to lift it free of the condyle. Sometimes this freeing does not occur and the horse is left with the leg straight, inflexible and extended as it tries to move off. Once the lock is freed, the horse moves quite normally until he again halts and relaxes.

There are two reasons why this condition may arise. When the horse is of upright conformation behind, the angles of the bones of the stifle joint, in relation to each other, mean that the patella ligaments catch on the femur. Alternatively, since muscle contraction is necessary to lift the patella clear of the condyle, poor muscling can be the cause. No

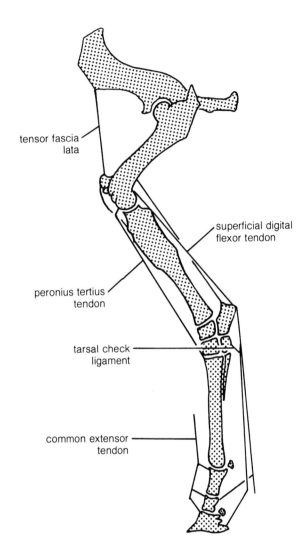

Fig 86   Ligaments supporting the left hind limb.

abnormalities can be felt in the joint. The condition is sporadic and distressing to both horse and observer when it occurs. However, the patella can often be freed by shouting or slapping the horse on the rump – the sudden increase in tension of the muscles will free the patella.

Where the horse's condition is poor, an improvement in muscling is often all that is

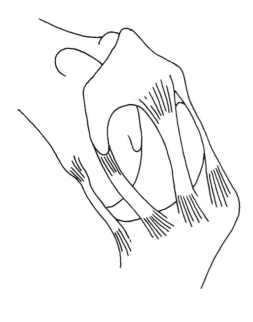

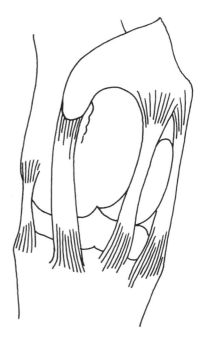

Fig 87   Topography of the stifle during movement.

Fig 88   Topography of the stifle in a resting position.

needed to cure the condition. If this is not successful, the patella ligament inside the leg can be cut surgically, so that the lock no longer functions. This procedure is easily performed, highly successful and immediately curative. Surprisingly, the horse can still doze standing up.

In the young Thoroughbred, two other conditions, namely osteochondritis dissecans (OCD) and subchondral bone cysts comprise the majority of stifle lamenesses. The two conditions appear to be closely related. OCD is a form of damage to the cartilaginous surface of the femur in the stifle joint and is often associated with roach back, as a conformational defect. Subchondral bone cysts are present as large holes in the bone of the condyle of the femur. Clinically they manifest as intermittent lameness at about the time when the horse is put into training (18 months to 2 years) and they may result from damage at the point of load bearing. Whereas OCD carries a hopeless prognosis, a high proportion of horses with bone cysts respond to a six-month period of rest. Those that do not can be treated surgically, by packing the hole with a bone graft.

It is possible to confuse the jerky gait that is produced by fixation of the patella with several other conditions.

Myositis

Where there has been damage to the muscles of the buttock, usually as a result of sliding to a sudden halt, tearing of the muscles may result. With time, fibrous tissue may be incorporated into the muscle tissue and later even bone may be produced. These materials have less elasticity than muscle, so movement is restricted. Consequently, the gait develops a sudden jerk backwards just as the foot reaches the ground. In mild cases deep massage is often sufficient to free the adhesions formed between fibres, but in more severe cases, surgical removal of the scar tissue may be required.

125

Stringhalt and Shivering

Contrary to the myositis just described, in stringhalt the jerky action occurs as the foot is lifted and it may be sufficiently severe to make the foot hit the belly. The cause of stringhalt is not clearly understood but it appears to involve the lateral digital extensor tendon of one or both hind legs. The cause may be damage to the tendon itself or to the nerve supply to it. The jerky action appears to be totally involuntary and is exaggerated when the horse is asked to rein back.

Surgical removal of part of the tendon mentioned nearly always results in a degree of improvement and some horses may recover completely. This is in contrast to the similar condition of shivering, in which the prospect of recovery is extremely bleak. Shivering usually affects both hind legs and the tail. It is a nervous disease, again accentuated when the horse is reversed, in which the horse jerks its foot from the ground and stands with it quivering in a flexed position, with the leg held away from the body, before returning to normal. The condition is usually progressive and no effective treatment is known.

Azoturia

Because during work the muscle masses of the hind quarters are required to produce enormous amounts of propulsive energy over a very short period of time, it is not surprising that when great demand is placed on an unprepared or unfit muscle, damage will ensue. This damage is known as 'tying up' or 'set fast' in mild cases, and azoturia, paralytic myoglobinuria or exertional rhabdomyolysis in more severe cases.

The condition is typically seen in horses who are stabled and exercised irregularly, and when exercise has been delayed but the full feeding regime maintained. As a result, the horse feels too enthusiastic and pulls excessively.

Clinically the horse develops profuse sweating, excessively rapid breathing and pain in the muscles over the loins and hind quarters. The muscles become tense and swollen. If urine is passed it may be discoloured and can vary from amber through the colour of claret to that of Guinness. This discoloration is a good, rough guide to the severity of damage, although biochemical tests on blood for the breakdown products of muscle are ultimately more reliable. In severe cases the horse will become unable to move as the affected muscles harden. Finally it will be unable to stand. This stage is virtually never reached, however, since the rider is able to detect abnormal gait at a much earlier stage. The hind limb stiffness is much more difficult to recognise in the early stages when the horse is being driven.

Muscle physiology To understand this condition, a basic knowledge of the physiology of muscle function is required. Muscle is comprised of fibres arranged in parallel bundles. The fibres are filaments which overlap and slide over each other when the muscle contracts, thereby shortening the muscle. The contraction is initiated by a change in electrical potential (current) across the cell membrane, which results from a change in the concentration of electrically charged particles of minerals, particularly sodium and potassium, on each side of the cell membrane. Calcium is also involved in this process.

The energy used is derived from several sources, the relative importance of each source depending on the speed at which the energy is required. The basic ingredient for supplying energy is glucose or its stored form, glycogen. Initially this is broken down to pyruvate. This can be done very quickly and does not require oxygen, so that when there is a sudden, unexpected demand on the system, energy can be quickly produced. The second stage of the process is much slower and does require oxygen. When the animal is worked hard, there is a sudden build-up of pyruvate, but this can be maintained only for a short period of time, for example, when a horse is running a sprint race.

When an excess of glycogen is present and the demand is very severe, when the horse is asked to take a heavy load at a high speed up a steep hill for example, the accumulated pyruvate is shunted into a biochemical cycle which finally produces lactic acid. Lactic acid is an irritant to muscle fibres, causing them to swell and burst. They then release myoglobin, the oxygen carrying component of muscle, comparable with haemoglobin in the blood. This is removed by the blood and filtered through the kidneys, appearing in the urine where it is responsible for the discoloration during azoturia.

In a similar manner, small particles of muscle tissue can be removed into the urine and account for the floccular (woolly) appearance sometimes acquired by the urine. Larger particles may become lodged in the kidneys, preventing urine from being filtered and when severe, this may prove fatal.

With rest and appropriate medical treatment, together with a rapid reduction in feed intake and a gradual return to work, the horse usually recovers with no further problems. However, the return to work must be gradual since there is a tendency for the condition to recur. There will be some scar tissue replacement at the site of the muscle damage and muscle wastage can result although this is often not visible.

Causes The cause of the problem has many component factors. The condition is more common in mares. It is also related to the period of time that the horse spends in its stable, without exercise, and on a diet too high in energy content. Hard food must be restricted in horses not being worked and built up slowly with the work.

The nature of the food may be relevant. Boiled barley and flaked maize are easily metabolised sources of energy which may be too readily available, so that excessive stores are accumulated too quickly. A dietary deficiency of vitamin E has also been blamed as a contributory factor.

The work required of the horse must also be taken into account. Heavy weights carried up steep hills at high speed vastly increase the amount of work done by the horse, and hence the amount of lactic acid produced. This is particularly relevant at the onset of exercise. It is essential to prime the muscles by thoroughly warming the horse before any real work is done. This applies whether the horse is going five miles or fifty. It is not sensible to argue that as you are going fifty miles, it is not fair to add to the horse's burden for a further fifteen to thirty minutes before starting, unless you are intending to go the first few miles at warming up speed. If the horse is going to have azoturia, it will be in the first few miles and at that stage it does not matter how far you were intending to travel.

'Tying up' and 'set fast' are terms usually applied to mild forms of azoturia, in which there is no urinary discoloration. In these cases, covering the loins with a blanket and gentle walking is often sufficient to ease the condition.

Occasionally similar muscular conditions can arise in which the symptoms are atypical; other groups of muscles may be affected and clinical noticeable signs may not occur until after exercise is completed. In these cases the transmission of mineral particles within the muscle may be at fault and assessment of the problem may require complex biochemical testing.

PELVIC LAMENESS

Lameness arising from the region of the pelvis – the structure that joins the hind legs to the spine – often causes a degree of lameness in both hind legs. Such lameness may be attributed to a 'bad back' by the inexperienced owner. Several conditions of the pelvis are seen occasionally. Although dislocation of the hip joint is very rare, due to the strong support around the joint, fracture of the pelvis is much more common after a traumatic incident involving the pelvis. The degree of lameness and severity of signs varies depending on the site of fracture. Accurate diagnosis can be difficult, requiring an extremely powerful X-ray machine. Treatment nearly always involves resting. Where the fracture is between the hip joint and the point of the hip, the prospect for recovery is much poorer.

Damage by redworm larvae in the major blood vessels may cause clots to form in the vessels to the hind legs. Where the vessel is completely blocked, acute lameness may result, usually shortly after the onset of exercise. The horse sweats profusely and shows evidence of considerable pain. The affected limb is cooler than its counterpart. The lameness is intermittent and when the obstruction in the blood vessel is only partial, signs can be confusingly variable. Successful treatment of such cases by medical means, to reduce the clot, has been recorded.

Another soft tissue injury of the pelvic area, particularly in heavier, middle-aged competitive horses, jumped at speed, is strain of the sacroiliac ligament which runs between the front of the pelvis and the part of the spine to which the pelvis is attached. There may be an initial period of acute lameness but subsequently there may be only intermittent lameness and poor performance, with lack of impulsion. This injury may be a highly significant cause of lowered performance in horses. The toe on the affected side is often dragged, the foot is moved in a diagonal, sliding action due to the stifle being rotated outwards. The signs are more exaggerated downhill. With time there may be muscle wastage on the affected side.

Treatment   Box rest for two to six months will result in complete recovery of more than

fifty per cent of all horses with soft tissue injuries of the pelvic region.

BACK INJURIES

Diagnosis of back injuries in the horse is very popular, largely because without the aid of sophisticated and expensive equipment, confirmation or rejection of the diagnosis may be virtually impossible. Although diagnosed too often, back problems undoubtedly arise quite frequently in competitive horses, causing loss of performance.

Evaluation of back problems is limited by a general lack of knowledge of spinal disorders in the horse. Diagnosis is not easily reached, due to the horse's size and difficulty in feeling the structures of the spine. Pain cannot easily be localised and is often low grade. Furthermore, some horses appear to be naturally sensitive to pressure on the back without necessarily having any underlying problem. Persistent, exaggerated response, with stiffness and dipping as the rider mounts, is referred to as 'cold back'. This condition usually resolves rapidly once the horse starts to move and it is unclear whether it indicates a current back problem or merely a temperamental problem. Further co-operation and more open discussion between the veterinary and chiropractic professions would undoubtedly be mutually beneficial but, more important, would be in the best interests of the horse.

Consideration of the horse's conformation may be helpful in reaching a diagnosis. Short-backed horses are more likely to suffer from bony lesions, whereas longer-backed horses with greater flexibility show more damage in muscle and ligaments.

Anatomy of the Spine

A thorough understanding of the basic functional anatomy of the spine is required to put

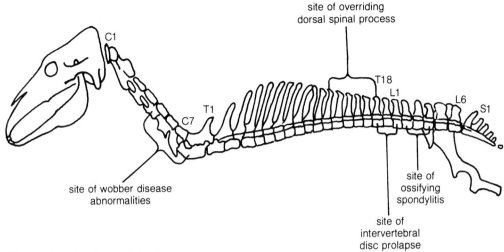

Fig 89 The vertebral column of the horse.

back problems into perspective. The spine consists of a series of 18 bony segments (vertebrae) over the chest or thorax, and 6 over the lumbar or abdominal area, each separated by thin intervertebral discs. These discs are composed of a strong, fibrous outer ring with a softer centre. The disc itself is immovable and when it becomes damaged, the outer ring bursts, allowing the soft central pulp to be squeezed out like toothpaste from a tube. If this material is squeezed into the spinal canal, it may apply pressure to the spinal cord causing partial paralysis. The process is not reversible, particularly since the area is surrounded by a mass of muscle.

To attempt to return the pulp would be similar to squeezing toothpaste back into a tube while the tube was surrounded by a boxing glove. Thus, to attempt to 'replace a slipped disc' suggests a complete failure to understand the pathology of the process. There is no evidence that such damage plays an important role in back injury in the horse.

The vertebrae are connected by a series of ligaments and muscles running longitudinally around the bones. In the centre of each is a bony canal through which the spinal cord runs, carrying vital nerves to the hind end of

the horse. Branches come off the spinal cord between vertebrae and supply the adjacent tissue.

There is very little movement in the spine along the thoracic and lumbar regions. The total vertical movement is approximately 5 cm. There is quite good movement between the last lumbar and first sacral vertebrae. The spine to the rear of the last rib allows no side to side or rotational movement. Consequently it is impossible to fulfil the demand of dressage tests that the spine be uniformly curved from head to pelvis. Virtually all curvature must take place in front of the shoulders.

Rising vertically from the arch (top) of the vertebra is a bony projection called the dorsal spinous process. This is quite long in the area of the withers and tapers to a squat process in the lumbar region. Projections can be felt individually along the middle of the back, particularly in the thin horse. In the mid-back, the spaces between these spines are narrowest and on occasions it is possible, when the back is dipped, for two or more processes to rub together, causing pain and loss of performance. This is particularly true in short-backed Thoroughbred-type horses. Such 'kissing', or overriding of dorsal spinous processes, needs

129

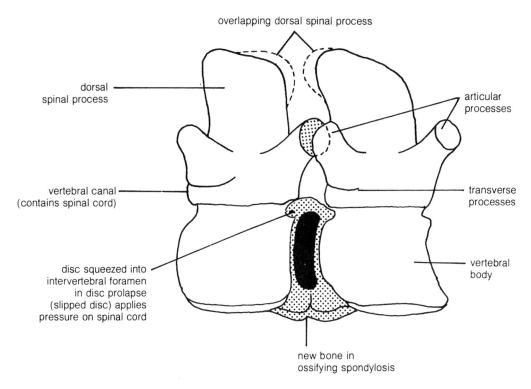

overlapping dorsal spinal process

dorsal
spinal process

articular
processes

vertebral canal
(contains spinal cord)

transverse
processes

disc squeezed into
intervertebral foramen
in disc prolapse
(slipped disc) applies
pressure on spinal cord

vertebral
body

new bone in
ossifying spondylosis

Fig 90 Diagrammatic topography of two adjacent vertebrae, to demonstrate the abnormalities arising in this area.

to be corrected by surgical trimming to prevent touching.

Bone damage to the vertebrae is not common. Ossifying spondylosis, the formation of new bone between vertebral bodies which is such a common problem in man, is rare in the horse. When it occurs, little can be done to alleviate the problem. Osteoarthritic changes on the transverse (side) processes and points where processes are attached are more common, but do not affect performance. Damage to the vertebral bodies usually follows a severe blow or fall and is dramatic in onset. Manual displacement of vertebral bodies, even after supporting muscle has been removed, is physically impossible. Animals are often said by chiropractors to have 'put out' or subluxated vertebrae and it is claimed that, by manipulation, such subluxations can be corrected. In fact, such manipulations cannot be performed,

even when all supporting tissue has been removed.

Most spinal problems result from damage to the muscles which support the spine, particularly the *longissimus dorsi* muscles on each side of the dorsal processes. When flexed singly, they are largely responsible (in conjunction with the elasticity of the intervertebral discs) for flexing the thoracic spine, but more importantly they work together to control the stiffness of the back during movement. During galloping and jumping they provide essential support to the backbone.

It has been suggested that vertebral subluxation is a misnomer, and that the irregularity in alignment along the spine results from local muscle injury, causing the muscle to go into spasm. The result is a slight curvature of the spine, affecting the pattern of locomotion. Manipulation of the spine may relieve the muscular spasm, producing at least temporary relief, or it may produce a similar, compensatory spasm on the opposite side of the spine.

The longer any curvature has been present, the more likely it is to result in loss of elasticity of the soft tissues on one side of the spine and therefore permanent curvature.

Treatment Treatment of back problems is not easy. Some conditions require surgical correction but in many cases a prolonged period of rest effects a spontaneous recovery. Often, however, six months or more is necessary.

The value of anti-inflammatory drugs is limited to the early stages of injury and in some cases a short course of treatment can be a useful diagnostic aid. Physiotherapy, particularly faradism, can be useful in cases of muscular injury. The principle is that small groups of muscle fibres can be made to contract individually using electrical stimulation. In this way, adhesions that may form between adjacent fibres can be broken or at least stretched, allowing the muscle action to return to normal. Swimming may also be helpful since the associated muscles can be exercised without the spine having to support the weight of the horse.

It should not be forgotten that back problems may be caused by poor schooling and equitation or a badly fitting saddle when there is loss of performance.

Spinal Cord Abnormalities

Fractures of the vertebral body associated with displacement will cause a degree of instability on usually two or more legs. In general, where the forelegs are involved, the injury is located in the neck or front of the thoracic spine. Mild cases may resolve spontaneously as the fracture heals, over a period of several months, but in severe cases the prospect for full recovery is usually hopeless.

Where onset of incoordination (ataxia) does not follow a traumatic incident, diagnosis can be very difficult. Examination of the spinal cord is not easy, particularly when the ataxia is only slight. It will be most marked when, as in dressage or show jumping, the horse is asked for precise coordination. A clinical neurological examination to decide which areas can feel pain and respond to stimuli is vital. Radiology can also be beneficial, but most machines are restricted to taking radiographs of only limited parts of the spine. Examination of blood for cell changes, presence of abnormal chemical substances or serological evidence of specific infections are all helpful.

In the young Arab or part-bred Arab, ataxia may develop at around four months, together with head tremors and a defective blink reflex. The cause is unclear but this breed may have a genetic susceptibility to a specific virus, causing degeneration of the cerebellum of the brain.

The young Thoroughbred may suffer from compression of the spinal cord at a specific point in the neck, as the result of a variety of deformities in the cervical vertebrae. These may follow rapid growth after excessive feeding. Although possible, hereditary connection has not been proven. Ataxia alone may be present, or it may be part of a complex clinical picture.

A variety of agents may infect the spinal cord, causing ataxia. Perhaps the most common is Equid Herpes Virus I (EHVI) which may cause hind limb ataxia and paralysis, particularly in mares. The severity may vary from slight dragging of the toes to a marked swaying and recumbency. Bacteria can cause infection in the bony vertebral bodies, or are the cause of abscesses round the spinal cord, but only in foals.

Damage caused by the larvae of redworms which migrate accidentally into the spinal cord is rare, as are tumours of the spinal cord.

11 Nervous System

The function of the nervous system is to co-ordinate the activity of each individual cell and organ with that of all other cells and organs so that the horse acts as an integrated unit. The system is necessarily extremely complex.

STRUCTURE

The basic unit is the neuron, comprising a cell body and processes (in some cases, extremely long ones) along which electrical impulses are transmitted. This is done by the movement of electrically charged ions (or mineral particles),

particularly sodium, potassium, calcium and chloride, across the cell membranes. Most neurons have many branches so that they can each communicate with many other cells. Between the individual cells are synapses across which electrical charges can pass in only one direction.

Anatomically the nervous system can be divided into the central nervous system and the peripheral nervous system. The spinal cord running along the back, protected by the neural arches of the vertebrae, forms the central nervous system. At the head, the spinal cord expands into the brain which accom-

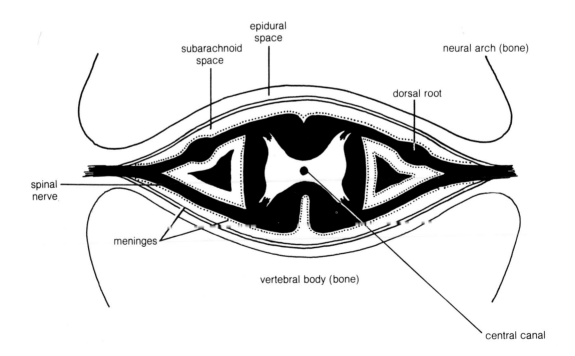

Fig 91 Cross-section through the spinal cord.

modates various specialised functions and co-ordinates activity from the whole body.

Running from the spinal cord are forty-two pairs of spinal nerves which form the basis of the peripheral nervous system, one pair for each body segment. The spinal nerves run out between the vertebral arches.

Functionally, the nervous system can be divided into somatic and visceral (or auto-nomic) nervous systems. The somatic nervous system relates to organs and tissues other than the gut and deals with voluntary muscle control and the sense organs. The visceral nervous system relates to involuntary control of large organs such as the heart and the digestive system, and the functioning of glands. Both these systems are present in the central and peripheral nervous systems.

Somatic Nervous System

The somatic nervous system accepts stimuli from the external or internal environment. The stimuli are analysed and produce the appropriate response. At its simplest, sensory nerve endings in or close to the skin, for example, respond to pain, heat, pressure or touch. They send messages by afferent sensory fibres *to* the spinal cord. The fibres synapse with efferent motor fibres which run *from* the spinal cord to the appropriate tissue, a muscle for example, causing it to produce the correct response. In this case, the system is a reflex arc. However, other fibres can travel to the brain so that the higher centre may affect the response. Similar sensory endings occur in tendons and joints so that tension and position can be appreciated by the horse.

Autonomic Nervous System

The autonomic nervous system is not under the control of the will. It is divided into two areas. The sympathetic nerves come off the spinal cord in the areas of the thorax and abdomen and run to the viscera. In general,

they are responsible for causing activity. The other areas, the head and the pelvis, supply the parasympathetic nerves. These generally suppress activity. Although branches do not originate in the chest or abdominal regions, branches extend from head and pelvis into these areas. Parasympathetic nerves in the vagus nerve from the head run to the heart, for example, controlling the intrinsic contractability of heart muscles.

PERIPHERAL NERVE ACTIVITY

Control

The nervous system can be likened to a river system, with a mass of tributaries running into larger streams which eventually all join a main river, in this case the spinal cord, running to an outlet (the brain). By damming the flow of impulses from the peripheral tissues to the spinal cord, it is possible to anaesthetise the area draining impulses through that point. Obviously the nearer the spinal cord that the damming occurs, the larger the area from which sensory impulses are lost. Such damming can be produced by a blow to the nerve, by surgical cutting of the nerve or by temporary infiltration of local anaesthetic around the nerve. Surgical sectioning of the nerve is carried out when a permanently painful lesion cannot be relieved in any other manner. This method has been used for the treatment of navicular disease. However, complications arise from the fact that the nerve supply to surrounding tissues is lost, so when any alternative treatment is available, it is likely to be preferable.

Temporary control of the transmission of pain impulses through nerves, using local anaesthetic, can also be useful in a variety of circumstances. In the lame horse, for example, where the cause of lameness is not obvious, the nerve supply to a specific area can be temporarily anaesthetised by strategic placing of local anaesthetic around that nerve. If the horse goes sound it can be assumed that the cause of lameness is within the area covered by that nerve supply. By starting at the foot and working up the leg, using various predetermined sites, the site of lameness can be localised. Although the results are not as clear-cut as might be expected, the technique can frequently be valuable.

Where it is unclear whether a lesion, for example a splint, is the cause of lameness, infiltration of local anaesthetic around the lesion can often provide the answer.

An alternative use for these techniques is to anaesthetise an area temporarily while carrying out a painful procedure. An area of skin can be infiltrated while a wound is stitched, or a nerve to the foot can be blocked while an abscess is drained. In cases where chronic pain is present as, for example, in cases of laminitis, the nerves to the feet can all be blocked using a long-acting, local analgesic or pain-killing drug. This will provide pain relief for five or six hours.

Damage

Damage to the peripheral nerves is usually manifested only as a loss of activity in that area supplied by the nerve or nerves involved. Usually the damage results from a blow where the nerve passes superficially over a bone. The condition is not painful since the pain detecting sensory nerves are also damaged. Initially there is local swelling in the area surrounding the nerve, and pressure on the damaged nerve causes loss of use. This pressure and bruising reaches a maximum after approximately twenty-four hours and then gradually subsides. There is then a slow return of nerve function, the duration of which depends on the severity of the initial damage, but frequently takes several months. Where three months have passed with no improvement in activity, further improvement is unlikely. If the initial

damage is caused by pressure resulting from a slowly enlarging tumour adjacent to the nerve, then the onset will be progressive over a much longer period of time.

A nerve which is vulnerable to damage from a blow is the facial nerve, where it runs across each side of the face to supply the ear, eyelid and lips. Usually only one side is affected and this results in the dropping of the upper eyelid and drooping of the ear on the affected side. Since the nerve supply to the muscles of the lips is damaged on one side, that side relaxes and the muzzle is pulled to the opposite side.

Damage to the nerves of the limbs results in a characteristic lameness in which the limb is dragged. There is no response to analgesic (pain-killing) drugs since the lameness is mechanical. Often the horse is simply unable to advance the limb beyond the vertical.

One condition which used to be far more common when draught horses were in use, was then known as Sweeny. This is a paralysis resulting from damage to the suprascapular nerve as it crosses the front border of the scapula or shoulder blade, before dividing to supply the two muscles on the outside of the scapula. Pressure from the harness collar would cause damage. Now a blow to the shoulder, often the result of a kick, will have the same effect. Often the first sign to be seen is that the spine or ridge on the scapula becomes prominent. This is because the muscles on each side of the spine – the supraspinatus and infraspinatus – shrink (atrophy) as a result of disuse. However, similar atrophy can occur when a horse is not using the leg as a result of chronic lameness originating somewhere else in the leg. Nerve damage in stringhalt and shivering is discussed in Chapter 10.

SPINAL CORD

Damage to the spinal cord will generally cause a loss of some or all functions posterior to the site of the lesion, depending on the severity of the damage. Such damage usually affects both sides of the horse, although not necessarily to the same degree.

Traumatic Injury

Traumatic injury to the spinal cord, from a severe fall for example, can result in failure of the reflex mechanisms which control the muscle tone in the tail, the neck of the bladder and the anus. Consequently the tail hangs limp and cannot be lifted up during defecation. The loss of faeces may also be uncontrolled. The bladder becomes distended with urine, and once it does so, urine overflows producing incontinence. In addition, there is likely to be a degree of paralysis or weakness in the hind limbs, ranging from an unsteady gait to complete inability to stand. Mentally the horse is alert and where the lesion is behind the shoulders the horse is quite strong on its forelimbs.

Other Factors

Besides trauma to the spinal cord, a variety of causes can produce similar signs of spinal cord damage.

Heredity Hereditary factors may produce a variety of lesions in the spine which result in compression of the cord and the 'wobbler syndrome'. Strictly speaking, this is a condition predominantly of the young male Thoroughbred with one of three recognised malformations of the vertebrae of the neck. The hereditary nature of the condition is complex and appears to be linked to the sex. The signs result from:

1. A constriction of the canal through which the cord runs.
2. Formation of new bone within the canal, causing pressure on the cord.
3. Instability of the vertebral bodies, allowing tilting and pressure on the cord above.

Onset usually occurs between birth and two years of age and is slow and progressive, often causing abnormality first in hind limb action and later in forelimb action. Severity of the signs depends more on the site of the lesion than on the degree of pressure on the cord.

The neck as the site of the lesion can be identified by checking the passage of nerve impulses along the cervical spinal cord. This is done by slapping the chest wall rhythmically behind the shoulder. Normally this will produce muscle contractions and movement of the vocal cords in the throat, which can be visualised using an endoscope inserted up one nostril. When there is damage to the cervical spinal cord, the response is absent.

Further diagnosis of the exact lesion is made using X-ray. The neck is not, however, a site which lends itself readily to radiography and the procurement of X-rays of diagnostic quality can be very difficult. The condition is usually not readily treated. Where there is instability of the vertebral body, screws between adjacent bodies can help to stabilise the lesion. This, however, raises the question of what should subsequently be done with the treated horse. The improvement is rarely good enough for the horse to be considered a trusted, safe ride. Furthermore, he cannot be used as a breeding animal, owing to the hereditary nature of his condition.

Infections Spinal cord lesions can also result from infections, either with bacteria or fungi, producing a meningitis. There is no specific cause of meningitis, which is far more common in foals than in the adult horse. Infection may enter through a penetrating wound to cause inflammation of the meninges or membranes surrounding the spinal cord. Usually the inflammation spreads to involve the brain, producing a meningo encephalitis. More often bacteria spread through the bloodstream from an infected navel in young foals, or from a strangles infection with *streptococcus equi*. Alternatively, fungi or misplaced wandering redworm larvae may produce similar signs. Meningitis is characterised by a general rigidity, increased nervous activity and so increased response to pain, excitement or depression and a raised body temperature. Treatment with antibiotics can be difficult, since it is necessary to find an appropriate antibiotic to combat the specific organism involved, and to find such an antibiotic which penetrates the spinal canal in adequate quantities.

Viruses may also cause spinal cord damage. In Britain, equine herpes virus can cause some damage, as can adenovirus, following the failure of the horse's immune system to combat its activity. The area involved is the *cauda equina* where the spinal cord finishes by dividing into a mass of individual fibres in the pelvic region, resembling a horse's tail. In adenovirus infection there is loss of muscle tone in the pelvic region, with wasting of the muscles over the hind quarters. Urinary retention with overflow is accompanied by retention of hard, dry faeces which produce a ballooning of the rectum. The condition is generally unrewarding to treat.

CONDITIONS AFFECTING THE BRAIN

Viral Infections

Most of the conditions which affect the brain result from trauma or the effect of toxins or poisons. Infections, both bacterial and viral, do occur but are relatively rare. In Britain, viral infections are not a problem. Rabies is the most common viral infection. Usually an infected horse is found dead, but when seen alive he can show a variety of clinical signs including limb paralysis, colic, muscle tremors or paralysis of the throat. At present rabies is absent from Britain and every effort should be made to ensure that this position remains.

Bacterial Infections

Bacterial infections can cause an encephalitis (inflammation of the brain) which has already been described with meningitis. The most common bacterial abnormalities of the brain result from the effects of toxins produced by the closely related bacteria *Clostridium tetani* and *Clostridium botulinum* causing tetanus and botulism respectively.

Tetanus

Tetanus or lockjaw is now more easily and more successfully treated than it used to be, but it is still extremely unpleasant, particularly since it can easily be avoided. The disease is surprisingly common and it is extremely unlikely that it will be eradicated since there is usually gross contamination of the soil on the ground inhabited by horses. Although all domestic species are affected by tetanus, the horse is particularly susceptible.

The spores of the causative organism may live in the soil for a number of years. When they become established in a suitable environment, they develop into active bacteria. As a result, they produce a poison or toxin which travels along the nerves to the spinal cord and then the brain. When the brain is intoxicated, clinical signs are seen. The site of entry dictates the period until signs develop. Hence a wound in the foot will take longer to develop signs than one in the neck. The period of development varies from a few days to several weeks.

Contrary to popular belief, large open wounds are not the most likely to become contaminated by tetanus organisms. Spores develop best in deep puncture wounds from which air is excluded, particularly if the blood supply is poor. Another favoured site is under a burn, where a superficial area of dead skin keeps the air from reaching the bacteria. In most cases of tetanus, however, the site of injury is not found and infection may have occurred through the intestinal wall. The bacteria can frequently be found in the dung of normal horses. This demonstrates the necessity of having a horse immunised against tetanus before it sustains a visible wound.

Symptoms The clinical signs consist of a slowly progressive paralysis of the muscles of the limbs, head and neck, and ultimately the respiratory muscles, so that death from asphyxia ensues.

Lockjaw is not a totally appropriate name for the condition in the horse since inability to open the jaw is a later development. The first signs are subtle, the most consistent being a protrusion of the third eyelid across the corner of the eyes. This protrusion is exaggerated if the horse is excited. The ears are pricked as the muscles at their base become paralysed. For the same reason, the dock of the tail is slightly raised. An anxious expression on the horse's

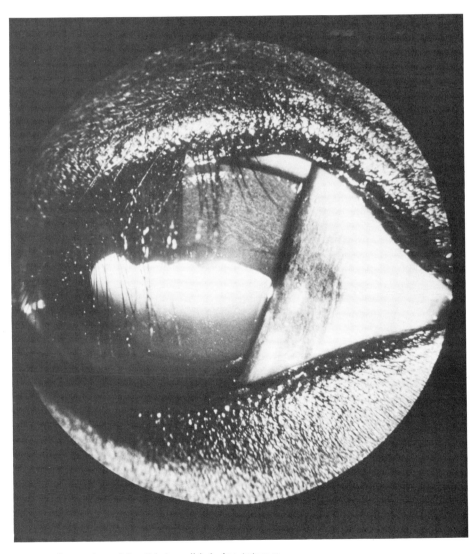

Fig 92   Protrusion of the third eyelid during tetanus.

face results from a spasm of the muscles to the corners of the mouth, drawing the lips back in a worried smile. At this stage the condition can be treated successfully.

Once this stage is reached, the disease develops rapidly and prospects for recovery become progressively more bleak. In the next phase, the legs become paralysed so that the gait becomes stilted and finally the horse develops a trestle-like appearance, unable to move its legs at all; if pushed, he will fall over with his legs still extended.

Treatment This is aimed at reducing muscle spasm. Because the animal is extremely excitable and excitement causes further muscle spasm and paralysis, the most important con-

sideration is the reduction of stimulation. This is best achieved by placing the horse alone in a darkened loose-box, keeping noise to a minimum and visiting him as little as possible. When his ability to eat or drink is lost, food and water must be supplied through a nasogastric tube placed in the stomach through the nose. This procedure may need to be continued for days or even weeks.

Medical treatment aims to kill the organisms producing the toxins and to neutralise the toxins. The bacteria are destroyed by thoroughly cleansing and aerating the wound wherever possible, and by using a suitable antibiotic. Neutralisation of the toxin acting on the nervous system is done using a tetanus antitoxin. The best results are obtained when

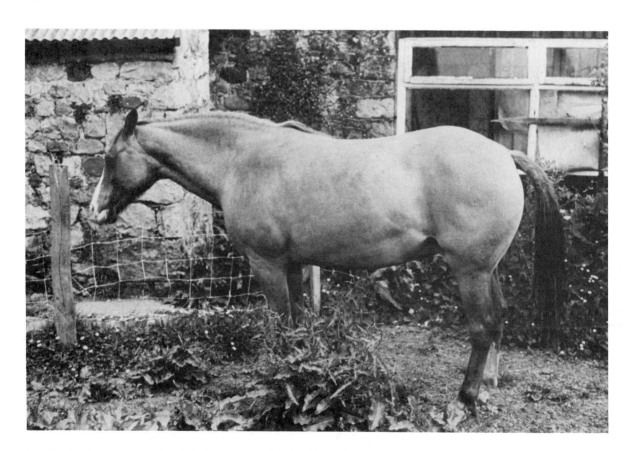

Fig 93 Tetanus – note the pricked ears, raised tail and paralysed tongue protruding.

antitoxin is introduced into the horse as near as possible to the site of action of the toxin. Consequently, when placed directly into the spinal canal, the maximum concentration comes into direct contact with the toxin.

There is often confusion over the difference between vaccination and the use of antitoxin. When a horse sustains an injury, tetanus antitoxin is given to neutralise any toxin that may be formed. This has an immediate, passive effect, but after approximately two weeks it is completely eliminated from the horse, who is then left unprotected. Vaccination involves the introduction into the horse of tetanus toxoid – a deactivated form of toxin which can do no damage but which stimulates the horse to develop its own immune system to destroy tetanus bacteria when they become established in the tissues. This development does not occur immediately. The first dose merely alerts the immune system and primes it. A second dose a month or so later stimulates a full-scale response by the horse, and over the next seven to ten days immunity gradually develops to a maximum. The immunity thus achieved lasts for a considerable time. Gradually the immune system 'forgets' about tetanus organisms and immunity wanes unless boosted by regular booster vaccinations, first after nine to twelve months, then at three-yearly intervals. In the pregnant mare, a booster given approximately one month before foaling will maximise the level of immunity provided passively in the milk, protecting the young foal until its own system has developed adequately to be stimulated by vaccination at four months old. It should be noted that vaccination cannot be given at the time of injury and be expected to provide protection for that injury.

When the treated horse recovers from the disease, he will have undergone considerable nursing and will remain physically weak for many weeks after resuming normal feeding and movement.

Botulism

Botulism is in many ways a similar disease to tetanus, but one which has only recently become a problem in Britain. Its appearance coincides with the feeding of 'big bale' silage to horses. The causative organism – *Clostridium botulinum* – again produces a toxin which affects the central nervous system. The toxin acts by preventing nerve impulses from passing to muscle fibres and so causes a progressive muscular paralysis and inability to stand.

Initially the affected horse is depressed but does not lose his appetite. However, paralysis of the tongue and throat prevent swallowing so that food is dropped back out of the mouth, giving the appearance of a tooth problem except that saliva is also drooled from the mouth. The next stage is progressive weakness of the legs and finally paralysis of the respiratory muscles. In contrast to tetanus where paralysis is spastic (that is, muscles become locked in spasm), in botulism paralysis is flaccid (loose and floppy) so that the limbs become totally relaxed. Mortality is high – up to 90 per cent.

Speed of progression of the disease depends on the dose of toxin taken in, death occurring after anything from a few hours to a week. Confirmation of the diagnosis is difficult since by the time the nervous system is affected, levels of toxin in the gut and blood are virtually undetectable.

Treatment This is essentially supportive nursing. The specific use of antitoxins as in tetanus cases, while being theoretically possible, is not economically practical. Furthermore, prevention by vaccination is not possible since vaccination works by stimulating the body to produce the means to kill the causal organisms. In botulism, the causal organisms proliferate outside the horse and the toxin is taken in through the feed. Clinical signs develop after approximately one week.

Prevention The clostridia thrive in an environment which is moist, not too acid, and free from air. A recent survey showed that 5.7 per cent of all soil samples contained the clostridia. Low levels of organisms often occur in the intestines of birds and mammals. The correct conditions for production of organisms are presented in large bales of silage, wrapped in plastic to exclude the air, particularly if the bales are not clean but contain soil or even animal material such as moles or pheasants picked up in the baling process. Wilting helps to increase the dry matter content and reduce the likelihood of contamination. Clamp silage has a higher level of acidity in which organisms cannot so readily reproduce; it is therefore safer to feed. Silage is becoming an increasingly popular feed for horses, both on economic and convenience grounds, and because it is healthier for horses with respiratory diseases. However, careful selection should be made, considering aroma (silage with low dry matter content undergoes secondary fermentation, producing a sour smell), dry matter content, acidity and whether the wrapping is intact. (This problem does not seem to occur with commercially bagged haylage)

Mineral Poisoning

Other toxic agents which commonly affect the central nervous system are either minerals or plant poisons. They, like the bacterial toxicities already described, affect both sides of the body equally and involve many nerves.

Lead poisoning Among the mineral poisons, only lead is seen with any degree of frequency. Even this is less common than it used to be, since one of the prime sources of poisoning was the chewing of objects painted with lead paint. Lead has not now been incorporated in paint for many years. The chewing of old car batteries lying in the field is another potential source of the toxin.

Lead is not broken down and can remain in a toxic state for many years. The peripheral nerves are affected in the same way as with botulism. Clinical signs are therefore similar and include paralysis of the throat, making swallowing difficult and producing a characteristic noise during breathing, since the vocal cords are paralysed. Subsequently there is muscular weakness in the legs. Affected horses often show a change in the red blood cells and lead can be detected in the blood and urine.

The lead can be removed from the blood by binding with a specific agent injected into the blood. This does not always produce any improvement, however, since it does not combine with the lead *within the cells* and it is this lead which is producing the clinical signs. Signs may suddenly develop some time after uptake has ceased, when the horse may not even have access to the source.

Plant Poisoning

Plant poisons can be difficult to differentiate by the signs they produce. The majority cause broadly similar symptoms which may include colic, acute diarrhoea, muscle tremors and convulsions. Hundreds of plants have been incriminated as being poisonous and merely finding a potentially poisonous plant in the pasture, even if it has obviously been grazed, does not confirm a diagnosis. A few plants do produce fairly specific clinical signs. Generally poisonous plants are not palatable but where food is scarce or where they cannot easily be sorted from a more palatable food (in hay, for example) they may be eaten. Very few plant poisons have specific antidotes and treatment is usually supportive. Prevention by controlling access to toxic plants is vital.

Ragwort Ragwort is one of the most common plant poisons. This produces severe central nervous signs which result from chronic cirrhosis of the liver. Toxic products produced in the damaged liver affect the higher centres of the brain, causing yawning, a sleepy appearance, pressing the head against a solid object or aimless wandering. Later the horse may stagger and behave dangerously. The liver damage is irreversible and intoxication usually ends in the destruction of the horse.

Bracken Bracken is also one of the plants more commonly causing toxicity. It is poisonous whether grazed fresh or eaten in hay. Toxicity is more common after a dry summer, when grass is in short supply. Onset is insidious, reflecting the intake of toxic material over a prolonged period. It shows first as a weight loss. Following this the gait becomes progressively unsteady with a hind limb weakness and the horse is unable to stand. This toxicity is one for which there is a specific antidote. The bracken contains an agent – thiaminase – which breaks down thiamine (vitamin B1). By supplying this vitamin, a rapid recovery can be achieved.

Foxglove Fresh foxglove plants are bitter and are therefore not readily grazed, but may poison hay. A horse would need to consume four or five ounces to show signs of toxicity. Again, one of the primary effects is to slow the heart since the parasympathetic nerves are stimulated. At the same time, stimulation of the sympathetic nerves causes diarrhoea. The slowing of the heart, with increased force of contraction, is used medically as a treatment of heart failure to improve heart activity. The toxic effect of digitalis, the active principle, is used at a carefully controlled level as a medical aid. Where this effect is carried to extreme, however, the result is circulatory collapse.

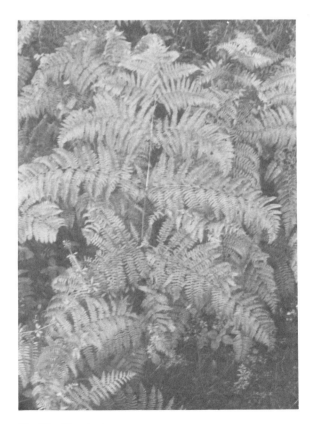

Fig 94 Bracken

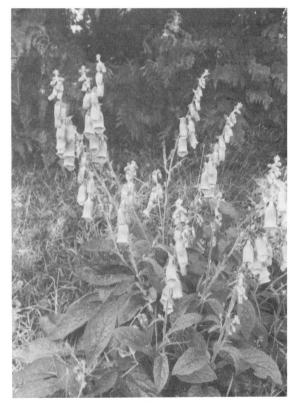

Fig 95 Foxgloves

141

Yew Yew, both the English and Irish varieties, are among the most toxic of plants. All parts are poisonous apart from the fleshy red cup around the seed. The toxic principle – taxine – is rapidly absorbed and poisons the heart, even in very small quantities. The action is so rapid that yew may still be present in the mouth of the dead animal.

Laurel The laurel is not normally eaten due to its leathery, indigestible leaves. It is as well that poisoning is rare since the leaves contain hydrogen cyanide which paralyses sensory nerve endings. Normally oxygen is carried in the blood by haemoglobin and when it reaches the tissues the oxygen is released to the cells. Cyanide combines with oxyhaemoglobin to form a stable compound so that the oxygen is not given up to the cells and the cells effectively suffocate. Furthermore, the heart muscle is poisoned directly and death results from cardiac and respiratory failures.

SYMPATHETIC AND PARASYMPATHETIC SYSTEM DISEASES

Grass Disease

One of the most commonly occurring enigmas of the autonomic nervous system is grass disease. This condition, originally restricted to the western seaboard of the United Kingdom, has gradually spread to cover virtually the whole country. Considering the intensity of research which the condition has provoked over fifteen years, little progress has been made. The jigsaw is gradually being completed, piece by piece, to try to provide the answers.

One of the problems which delays progress is that the disease takes a variety of forms although with a few common features. Furthermore, diagnosis can be confirmed only by post mortem, and then not easily. The signs that are

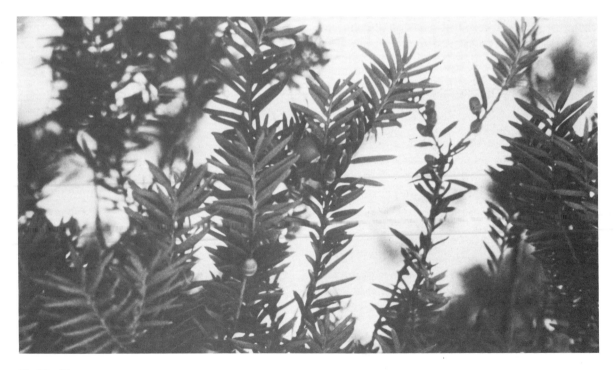

Fig 96   Yew

produced are easily confused with colic produced from a variety of causes. There is not a predisposition in terms of age or sex or breed, but the disease is confined to grazing animals and occurs in ponies more frequently than in horses, although this may reflect the fact that more ponies are grazed. It occurs more frequently in the period May to July, particularly during dry weather or during a cold, wet period following warm and sunny weather. Another high risk group of horses is young mares who are about to foal and have travelled to new premises. Both of these two factors may indicate increased stress on the animal.

Symptoms The signs of disease vary from the extremely acute, with death occurring in two or three days, through a spectrum to chronic cases showing gradual wasting over a period of weeks or months. The more acute cases show signs of severe colic, regurgitation of fluid stomach contents down the nose, and paralysis of the throat. The muscles tremble in an uncontrolled manner. Initially there may be diarrhoea, but later no dung is passed and on examination the faeces are found to be hard and black. In less severe cases, death follows approximately three weeks of dull abdominal discomfort. Again, stomach contents are returned down the nose and the dung is hard and dry. When observed, the horse stands with a dipped back and the feet brought together under the body. In the more chronic cases, where gradual wasting follows recurrent regurgitation of stomach contents, small quantities of soft cow-like faeces may be passed.

All the signs reflect inactivity of the gut and although the large intestine contains hard, dark faeces, the fluid content of the small intestine may be up to three times the normal level.

It is generally accepted that in this condition the nervous stimulation of the gut activity is interrupted. Evidence to support this comes from characteristic changes found in certain areas of the autonomic nervous system. The nervous system of the gut is complex and changes in a basic regulatory protein, which controls gut contractions and production of fluid secretions into the gut, are thought to be responsible. However, there is a further complication, since it is possible to transmit these changes experimentally from one affected horse to an apparently normal horse, and reproduce the changes, without the horse showing clinical signs of the disease. A trigger factor must also be involved to trigger the clinical condition.

The search is on for some factor, possibly a plant poison or a virus, which produces the pathological changes in the nervous system and a second trigger, possibly stress, which produces the clinical disease. Travel or change in temperature or environment are known to increase significantly sympathetic nerve activity and may be responsible for the signs of sweating, muscle tremors and rapid pulse. This increase in activity may, however, be a cause or an effect of the disease and much work needs to be done to reach a satisfactory conclusion.

VICES

Vices encompass a wide range of mild and more serious habitual, atypical behaviour, which may include kicking in the stable, aggressiveness, destructiveness of the surroundings or pawing. It is important to differentiate these vices from temporary behavioural changes where an underlying cause may be present. For example, pawing may be a sign of a mild abdominal pain. Disturbances in sexual activity, particularly in mares, may result in displays of uncontrollable temper, or changes in temperament may reflect ill treatment in the past. It is as well to remember that it is the duty of a vendor to disclose that these vices are present when a horse is sold.

Crib Biting and Wind Sucking

Much confusion arises in the terminology used to differentiate these vices. 'Grasping' is the state in which a horse may hold a fixed object between its incisor teeth, sometimes as a sequel to licking it. The crib biter or 'cribber' uses the fixed object which it has grasped to flex and arch his neck and pulls back so that pressure is applied to the upper teeth. No air is swallowed. To do this, the horse will hold the manger, stable door, gate or fence post but in the absence of these, considerable ingenuity is shown, using the knee, for example.

When the horse goes on from this state to swallow air, usually with a characteristic grunt, it is recognised as a wind sucker. Wind suckers may not need to grasp an object to swallow air. They may rest their incisors on a fixed object without grasping it or they may rest their chin on an object and swallow air. Alternatively, wind sucking may be performed with no fixed object at all. Wind sucking may follow crib biting when the horse is prevented from cribbing.

Crib biting is considered undesirable for several reasons. It often results in damage to property although this is not nearly as extensive as that produced by horses which are fence chewers. There is erosion of the incisor teeth which may be extensive and result in dental disease. There will also be excessive development of the sternocephalicus muscle on the underside of the neck, where the neck is

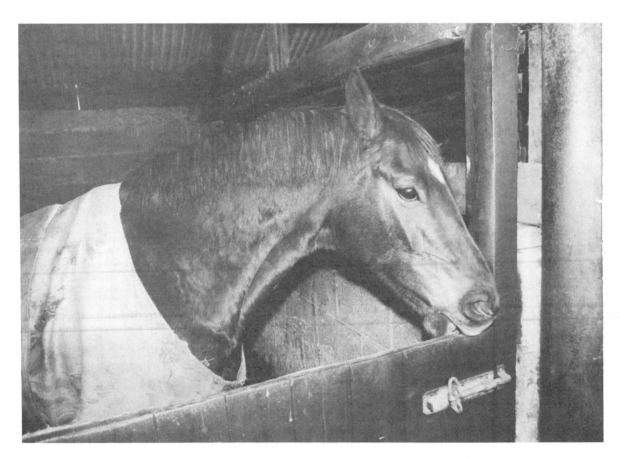

Fig 97   Using the stable door to crib bite.

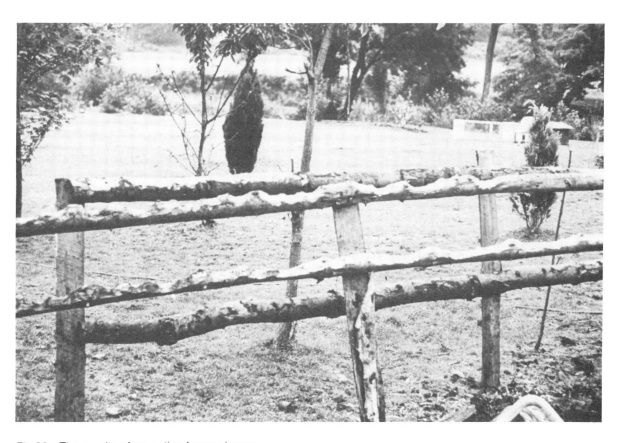

Fig 98   The results of an active fence chewer.

continually flexed. Furthermore, there is often a fear that the habit will be passed on to other horses in the same yard, although as will be seen later, this is improbable. Horses that swallow air are unable to eructate that air easily, so it continues through the gut to be produced as flatus. This process often causes abdominal discomfort and may lead to flatulent colic. The horse also shows poor performance and weight loss.

The cause of these vices is unknown. Originally gastritis was thought to be the cause and that by swallowing air the horse obtained relief. There is no evidence that affected horses have any such affliction. Boredom is also unlikely to be the cause; the incidence would be higher in horses which are inadequately exercised and relatively overfed, which is not

the case. The habit is often seen when the horse is moved to a strange environment, although no suggestion of a vice has been present before. In these circumstances, boredom should be least likely. The vice may even develop in the first few weeks of life, when boredom is extremely unlikely.

Crib biting is most frequently carried out when the horse is feeding. The habit is absent from horses in the wild or even from wild horses brought into captivity; these suffer from boredom more than the domesticated horse. Crib biting does not occur as a result of imitation, although it must be remembered that the same trigger factors may be presented to several horses in the same yard. The vice seems to be a natural trait, more prevalent in certain breed lines and triggered by some

145

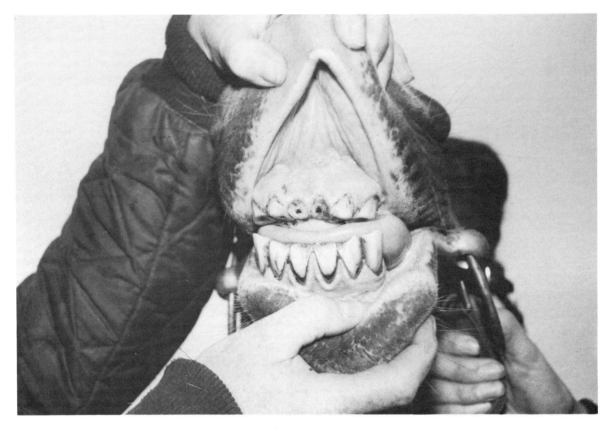

Fig 99   Erosion of the incisor teeth after crib biting.

unidentified factor. The incidence seems to be greater in horses with a nervous disposition.

Treatment   Correction of the habit is approached along four lines.

1.   Prevention of grasping, by removal of suitable edges, or the use of a muzzle. Edges can be rendered unsuitable by making the edge of the manger too wide or by fixing guttering to the top of the manger or stable door. Feeding from a manger on the ground may be helpful since the horse can not flex his neck while eating from the ground. The horse does not, however, grow out of the habit and as soon as he is presented with the opportunity, will resume the vice.

2.   The second approach is to make grasping unpleasant. This is done either by smearing appropriate surfaces with preparations which taste unpleasant – aloes, blister or creosote – or by the use of an electric wire. The latter is useful in a limited number of cases, but horses will learn to tell when the wire is live by listening for the click of the battery as the current is passed.

3.   A strap applied to the gullet may prevent arching of the neck. Occasionally a simple leather strap is sufficient, but more commonly a gullet plate is used, so that when the neck is arched the horse is unable to swallow. Alternatively a cribbing strap can be used. This strap has a ring of metal prongs which are sheathed in the strap. When the neck is arched the prongs are forced out of the collar and apply pressure on the throat.

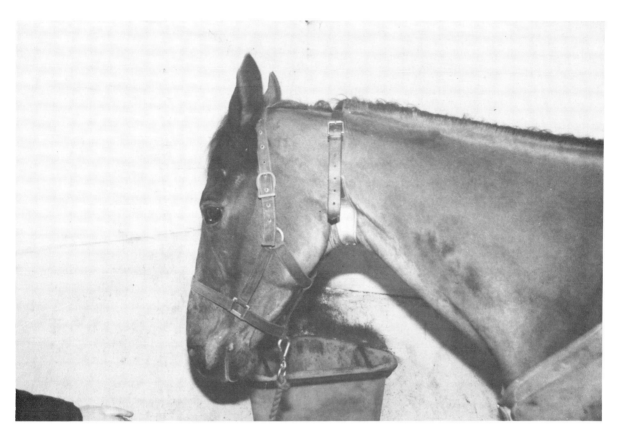

Fig 100   The use of a gullet strap (cribbing strap) to prevent crib biting.

4.   Finally surgery can be used. Most surgical techniques are based on those developed by Forssell early in the century. They involve removal of portions of the muscles of the neck so that the horse is incapable of flexing it. This operation has approximately 50 to 60 per cent success rate in the short term, but is less successful in the long term. Frequently horses will start the vice again within a few days of surgery.

A cosmetically more pleasing alternative is to remove the nerve supply to the muscles but, since the muscles have collateral nerve supplies, the success rate is poor. A combination of removing the nerve supply, together with small amounts of muscle, seems to be the most successful compromise, producing the success rate of Forssell without the extensive, dis-figuring, surgery.

Contrary to expectation, the sectioning of nerves is more effective in controlling the swallowing of air than in controlling crib biting.

Since a vacuum is necessary in the mouth for horses to swallow air, a technique of making holes in the sides of the cheeks (buccal fistulae) is effective in preventing the swallowing of air. However, leakage of food and saliva through the holes makes the procedure unpleasant. Furthermore, it is difficult to prevent the holes from sealing over spontaneously.

Weaving

Weaving is a nervous habit seen in a variety of animal species and arising from boredom. The horse rocks from side to side as it moves its head, shifting its weight from one foreleg to the other. This habit is rapidly copied by other horses and so means that the weaver must be kept apart from other horses. The movements increase in prominence before feeding, urination or defecation.

Treatment Weaving can be reduced by using vertical bars above the stable door to prevent sideways movement. An alternative that has been suggested is to suspend heavy weights level with the horse's head in front of the box, so that as he moves sideways he will hit his head.

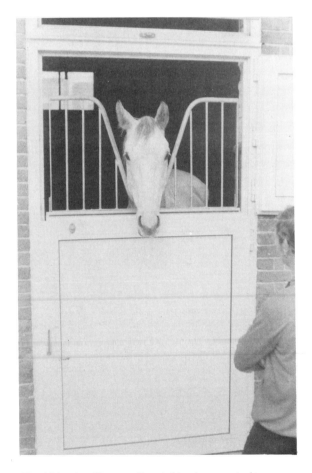

Fig 101 A grille over the stable door controls weaving effectively.

Head Shaking

Head shaking appears to be a syndrome rather than a specific condition. That is, it is a collection of signs which may be caused by a variety of factors, some of which can be identified but a large proportion of which cannot. The condition is characterised by involuntary vertical jerking of the head as though in response to an irritation on the nose. Usually it is present solely, or more frequently, in warmer, humid weather and usually in strong sunlight. It occurs most frequently in horses who are being ridden and can become so severe that it makes riding dangerous; however, more severely affected horses may head shake at any time.

It is reasonable to assume that the phenomenon is in response to irritation in the head area and, indeed, in a proportion of horses this proves to be the case. Ear mites, deep in the horizontal canal of the ear can cause this problem. Occasionally the signs follow diseases of the sinuses which may occur following abnormalities in the cheek teeth roots.

It has been suggested that the problem results from too-heavy hands riding a light-mouthed horse, but this does not explain its seasonal incidence, nor the horses who head shake when not being ridden. The underlying cause in most cases appears to be an allergic inflammation in the nose, in response to many allergens from pollens, and possibly from trees or nettles. Most affected horses have some signs of allergic lung disease.

Treatment Some horses respond favourably when moved to a completely new location. Two approaches to treatment may be made.

1. An inhalant steroid can be used to reduce inflammation. This involves applying an inhaler for two to five minutes before the horse is ridden. Besides being inconvenient, this would

not be allowed before competitive riding.

2. A quite effective remedy, at least temporarily, is to cut the infraorbital nerves so that the nostrils become desensitised. This does, however, have a drawback, since horses use their sense of touch at the nostrils for guidance and following desensitisation can become seriously disorientated, particularly at night.

Perhaps physical attempts to correct vices are not a suitable approach. An attempt at correcting the environmental factors which trigger these phenomena is likely to prove more fruitful in the long term. Crib biting and wind sucking may result from a desire to eat for longer periods, and to fill the stomach with greater bulk – both features of the naturally grazing horse. By rendering the food more difficult to eat, perhaps by providing a hay net with smaller holes, it may be possible to reduce weaving. Likewise, the use of extruded concentrates in the diet may be useful; these are concentrates mixed with water and air and squeezed through a nozzle. This process makes them harder to chew. They increase the feeding time and the bulk of food in the stomach and reduce the desire of the wind sucker to supplement it with air.

12 Urinary System

The organs of the urinary system are the kidneys, ureters, bladder and urethra. The kidneys of the horse are situated on either side of the spine, tucked against the dorsal wall of the abdomen. They weigh about 700g each and are held in place by the pressure of the surrounding organs and by the renal fascia, a specialised sheet of connective tissue which encloses both kidneys. Each kidney is connected to the bladder by a tube called a ureter. Ureters arise from an area of the kidney called the renal pelvis and pass from there to the bladder, their function being to transport urine from the kidneys to the bladder.

When it is empty the bladder is about the size of a clenched fist and it lies on the floor of the pelvis. The stored urine passes from it to the exterior through a long tube called the urethra.

KIDNEY STRUCTURE AND FUNCTION

Internally, the kidney consists of many units called nephrons. These begin with a structure known as the glomerular capsule and pass as a looped tube through the body of the kidney to a series of collecting tubes. These ducts then empty into the renal pelvis which in its turn empties into the ureter.

In excreting urine, the kidney is the main regulator of blood plasma composition. It excretes nitrogenous waste products in the form of urea, removing excess water and inorganic salts from the body system and also any foreign substances that may have gained access to that system. It does this by a process of filtration and selective reabsorption. As the blood passes through a complex system of capillary loops in the glomerular capsule, water and plasma constituents are filtered out into the renal tubule. As the plasma-like fluid passes down the tubule, those salts and water that the body needs are reabsorbed. What is left passes down the tubules into the renal pelvis and is excreted as urine through the ureters and urethra.

DISEASES

The horse, in comparison with other species, suffers few diseases of the urinary system. Three conditions that do occur are:

Urinary Calculi

Urinary calculi (stones) are collections of mineral salts which form around a nucleus of organic material. They can be found anywhere in the urinary tract, but reach their largest size in the bladder. Two types of calculi are formed. One, high in calcium salts, is found in horses fed on a diet high in hay or grass. The other type is high in phosphates and is found in horses being fed on a predominantly grain diet.

Horses suffering from urinary calculi show a variety of symptoms depending upon the position of the stone. Discomfort whilst urinating, abdominal pain and increased frequency of urination are common signs. Blood in the urine or the passing of blood clots may be seen. Rectal examination may confirm the diagnosis. Treatment is generally by surgical removal of the stone, although the use of smooth muscle relaxants can relax the urethra enough to permit the passage of small stones.

Cystitis

Cystitis is an inflammation of the bladder. In the horse it is generally secondary to other conditions such as urinary calculi or vaginal infection. Injury to the urethra and bladder following foaling can also cause cystitis.

Frequent urination is a common symptom. The quantity of urine passed is small and the horse frequently stands with legs straddled for some time, attempting to pass more. Urination is obviously painful and the urine is thick, cloudy and contains pus and clots of blood. Bacteriological examination will demonstrate the wide range of bacteria which can cause cystitis.

Once the primary cause of cystitis has been removed, the secondary infection can be treated with a wide range of antibacterial drugs.

Renal Disease

Primary nephrosis 'degeneration of the kidneys' and nephritis 'infection of the kidneys' are rare in the horse.

Nephrosis is found secondary to many diseases. The toxins from acute infections, plant and chemical poisonings and viral infections can all cause a degeneration of the kidney tissue. The symptoms are often obscured by the signs of the primary disease. If the kidney damage is not too extensive and the horse lives, then the kidney regenerates.

Nephritis in the horse is seen as a complication of joint ill and foal septicaemia. Multifocal abscesses develop in the substance of the kidney. They are extremely resistant to treatment and the condition is unlikely to resolve.

13 Wounds and Injuries

The horse, of all the animals, is the most prone to injury. His surprising clumsiness in small spaces and his tendency to escape real or imaginary danger by uncontrolled flight, ensure that accidents will happen. Whether the accident is a cut in the skin or a penetrating wound, a strain to a tendon or a broken bone, the healing process is the same and a knowledge of how this process works is a necessary prerequisite to an understanding of treatment.

THE HEALING PROCESS

In all but the least of injuries, haemorrhage is the first step in the healing process. Blood leaks from the broken blood vessels into the damaged area and quickly clots, thus sealing the defect. At this stage the clot consists of fibrin – the body's Superglue – and both red and white blood cells. Within a few minutes an inflammatory process starts. The local blood vessels enlarge in size and flood the area with fluid, causing a local swelling. White blood cells, the defenders of the body, migrate into the area and start to digest the clot and any foreign material that might be present. As this process, known as phagocytosis, continues, the damaged area starts to shrink.

Skin

In the healing skin wound, epidermal cells (that is, cells from the skin margin), follow the white blood cell invasion and quickly form a new layer of skin under the superficial scab. In wounds where the edges are close together, such as a surgical incision, this occurs in 24–48 hours, but obviously it takes much longer in the larger wound. This single layer of cells takes about a week to grow and spread into a layer of fragile but complete skin.

The same process takes place in the depths of the wound. Cells called fibroblasts, normally found in connective tissue (the layer of tissue that connects skin to underlying organs) start to multiply. They migrate into the defect from the sides, moving along the strands of fibrin at about a tenth of an inch a day. In the typical surgical wound they meet in the middle in about a week.

Closely following the fibroblasts are a group of cells which originate from the small blood vessels at the edge of the wound. The endothelial cells, as they are called, multiply to form branching buds of tissue which burrow their way across the defect, again following the fibrin strands. This tissue quickly becomes canalised, allowing blood to pass into the defect, and by increasing the supply of healing agents, accelerates the healing process.

Thus, in a few days, the original blood clot becomes highly vascular (rich in blood supply), quickly growing connective tissue, a tissue known as granulation tissue. In the horse, granulation tissue often becomes an embarrassment as it overflows the boundaries of the defect and by its exuberant growth, prevents the development of new skin across the injury. In these cases the granulation tissue is known as 'proud flesh'.

As time goes on, the fibroblasts lay down a tough fibrous tissue called collagen. The blood vessels decrease in number as the collagen fibres increase, the white blood cells disappear and as the collagen contracts, the wound gets smaller and the repair stronger. Eventually, elastic fibres replace some of the collagen, making the wound more pliable and feeling returns as nerve fibres grow into the scar. The

152

wound is now effectively completely healed.

Bone

Bone heals in much the same way. Following a fracture, the large blood clot that forms at the fracture site is rapidly organised into granulation tissue, in this case known as a soft tissue callus. Over the next few days, cells from the bone margins, known as osteoblasts, together with fibroblasts, start to lay down a framework of cartilage and bone which immobilises the fracture. With time the callus reacts to the stresses of weight and muscle power and is remodelled by the laying down and reabsorption of new bone. If the realignment of the fracture was correct and the original stresses reapplied, almost perfect repair occurs.

Tendons

Unfortunately, the same cannot be said for the repair of tendons. Although the same principles govern the repair of tendons, the end results are often not as good. Tendon is comprised of bundles of collagen. They are organised in a plane parallel to the line of stress, as it is in this arrangement that they can withstand the most force. When the tendons of the horse are severed or ruptured, in particular the long, flexor tendons of the limbs, healing takes place, but the strong parallel arrangement of collagen fibres is not duplicated. Instead, a disorganised bundle of collagen results. This is not as strong as the original and frequently breaks down when put under strain; witness the large number of broken down racehorses.

WOUNDS TO THE SKIN AND SOFT TISSUES

Skin wounds are the most common injury that we see in the horse, and it is important to realise that they can heal in two different ways. The preferred way is healing by 'first intention',

that is, where the edges of the wound are held in apposition and quickly stick together. Healing by 'second intention' is a much longer process and occurs when the edges of the wound are apart, either because loss of tissue means that the edges cannot be joined or because infection or movement of the wound causes a breakdown. Healing of the wound must then wait until the gap between the edges of the defect is filled with granulation tissue. Only then can the skin grow over the surface. In some cases, 'proud flesh' develops, as mentioned above, and delays healing. Small amounts of proud flesh can be removed with chemical agents – copper sulphate in particular – but this method has the disadvantage of discouraging skin growth as well. Large areas of proud flesh require a different approach. In these cases skin grafts, using skin from other sites on the same horse, can be used. Perhaps the simplest technique is pinch grafting in which small pieces of skin, a few square millimetres in area, are removed, usually from the neck, and planted at approximately 1cm intervals over the site. The aim is for these pinches to form islands of new growth which individually spread out and cover the wound.

In practice, only about 30 per cent of grafts 'take' and often they fail to spread. However, the graft still performs a useful function as in these cases the proud flesh is suppressed by chemicals produced by the graft, allowing the skin margins to cover the wound.

Sometimes, following a blow or kick, the underlying tissues are damaged but the skin itself is unbroken. This type of injury, called a bruise, heals with very little trouble. Cold water compresses will, by reducing the swelling and inflammation, hasten recovery. If the damage is more severe and bleeding occurs under the skin, then a blood blister (haematoma) forms. The pressure of the escaping blood lifts the skin away from the underlying muscle. When the skin tension around the haematoma equals the pressure of the blood escaping, the bleeding stops and the haema-

153

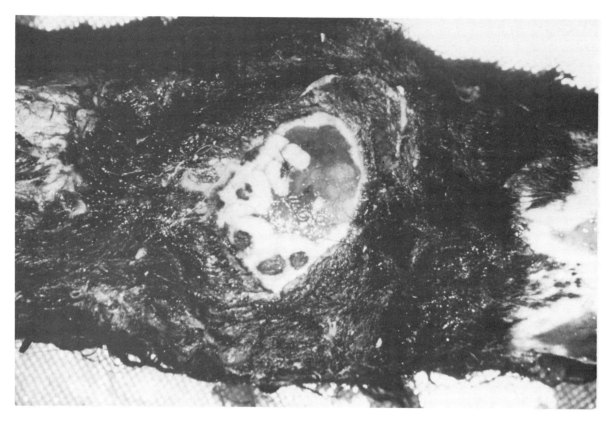

Fig 102   Pinch grafts slowly covering the wound surface.

toma stabilises. Once the blood in the haematoma clots, the plasma can be drawn off. The rest of the clot is then reabsorbed by the body.

Healing – Influences and Complications

1   The initial haemorrhage must be controlled. Too much bleeding prevents the initial healing process. Small cuts and grazes are no problem, as the severed veins and arteries quickly contract and cease bleeding, but larger vessels can bleed for some time and the haemorrhage should then be controlled by the application of a pressure bandage or, in extreme cases, with a tourniquet. If a tourniquet is applied, it must be released every quarter of an hour to ensure that circulation is maintained.

2.   A clean wound is important, as any contamination delays healing. Bacteria thrive in dirt and as they multiply, they and the toxins that they produce increase the damaged area and cause a delay in the time taken to cleanse the wound. Swabbing or syringing the area with a large quantity of warm, disinfectant solution will remove most of the debris. Larger particles can be removed manually. When the wound is dry and clean apply an antibiotic spray or solution and cover the wound with a clean dressing, either to heal on its own or to await further attention. At this stage do not use one of the many healing ointments or oils that are available. They are almost impossible to remove if at a later time your vet decides to stitch the wound.

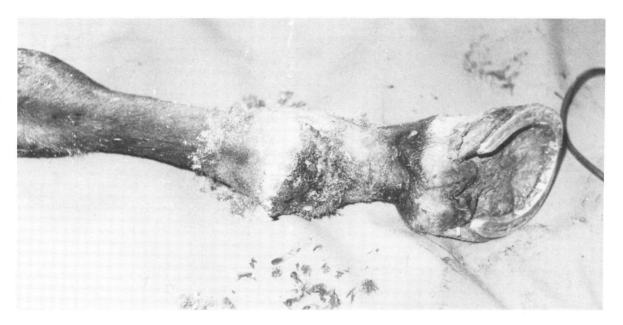

Fig 103   This type of wound must always heal by second intention.

3.   Excessive swelling, especially in wounds that have been stitched, is a frequent complication. The swelling that often accompanies wounds to the lower limb increases the tension on the suture line and thus increases the chance of a wound breakdown.

4.   Beware of the penetrating wound, especially the nail that pierces the sole of the foot. It is almost impossible to be sure that there is no foreign material in the depths of the wound. As these wounds are impossible to clean adequately, they need poulticing, to draw any dirt out, and antibiotics should be given to control the inevitable infection. All horses should be adequately protected against tetanus.

5.   Air is sometimes sucked into a wound by the pumping action of the body movement. Wounds in the armpit and behind the shoulder, generally caused by a penetrating stake, are particular offenders. The air spreads along under the skin causing a most alarming bubbling effect. Once the entry of more air is prevented, however, either by suturing the wound, or plugging the hole, the remainder is soon absorbed by the body.

6.   Wounds involving joints are potentially more serious. Each joint is enclosed by a tough capsule. If this is penetrated, the integrity of the joint is jeopardised. Synovial fluid (joint oil) continually escapes from the joint into the wound, delaying healing. Infection can enter through the break and cause a septic arthritis. This type of wound needs prompt treatment. If possible, the joint capsule should be repaired and the wound kept clean to minimise the chance of infection.

7.   As has been explained earlier, the closer the edges of a wound can be kept together, the quicker the wound will heal. The edges of small wounds can be joined by bandaging or by the use of sticky plaster, but larger wounds, especially those penetrating into the deeper layers of the body, require stitching or suturing. A sedative and local anaesthetic or, in the more complicated wound, a general anaesthetic, may be needed. The veterinary surgeon then repeats much of the work that has already been done. The haemorrhage is controlled, in

this case by clamping off the bleeding vessels. The wound is then thoroughly cleaned and any dead or damaged tissue removed, a process known as debridement. Often the wound is of such a shape that a pocket forms on the lower edge. Blood and fluid, dirt and bacteria collect in this pouch; they must be removed and the pocket obliterated before the wound can be stitched. If necessary, the underlying layers of tissue are brought together and held in place with sutures and finally the same is done with the skin.

Factors affecting first intention healing
The position of the wound is very important. Wounds parallel to the lines of strain, such as vertical wounds on the leg, heal much better than wounds that are at right angles to the lines of strain. Wounds above the knee and hock heal well, but those below do not. The lack of

underlying tissue, the poor blood supply and the excessive movement of these lower limb wounds inhibit satisfactory healing.

Wounds in which much skin and underlying tissue have been lost are a poor risk. In order to join the edges, considerable tension must be applied to the stitches and this excessive tension inevitably leads to a wound breakdown.

Finally, wound infection always causes a failure of first intention healing. A clean wound, with minimal damage is of paramount importance if that ideal, first intention healing, is to be attained.

BONE FRACTURES

For too long, the reaction to many cases of bone fracture has been immediate euthanasia of the horse. This need not happen. New tech-

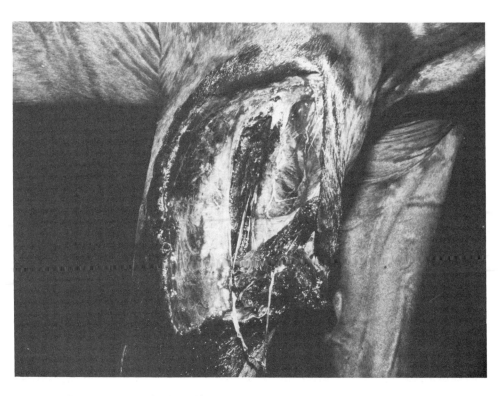

Fig 104 Even wounds as bad as this can heal well. This one took four weeks.

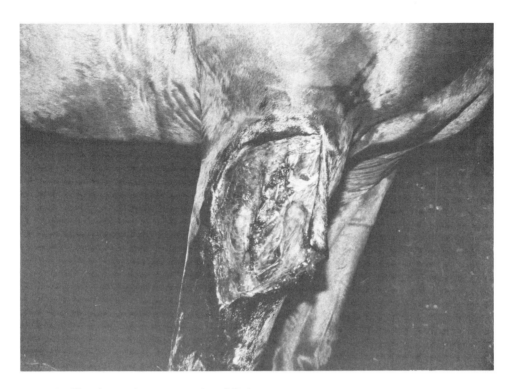

Fig 105   The deeper layers are sutured first.

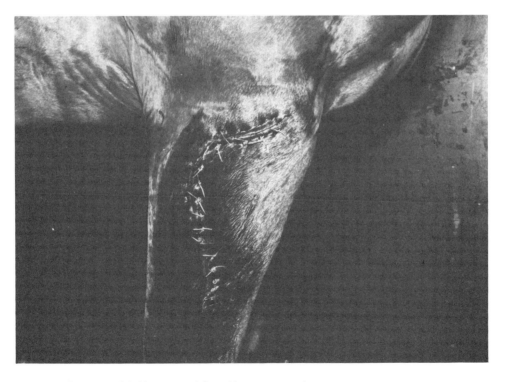

Fig 106   The superficial layers and the skin are sutured.

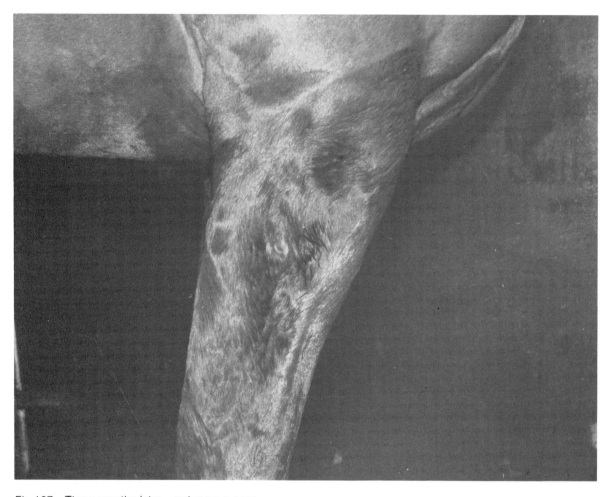

Fig 107   Three months later - not even a scar.

niques and stronger surgical materials mean that many fractures of the lower limb can now be satisfactorily treated and the horse returned to normal function. However, the surgical treatment, the materials and the after-care are expensive. All the more reason that adequate insurance cover is taken out. Fractures of the spine and upper limb are less likely to recover, except in the young foal, with little expectation of a return to full function.

The first step in the treatment of any fracture is accurate diagnosis. With such a diagnosis, an estimate can be made of the likely outcome of the case and its cost. The use of a Robert Jones splint or one of the new vacuum splints, together with painkilling drugs will allow most cases to be transported, with very little risk of further damage, to a hospital where X-rays and other diagnostic techniques can be undertaken. A Robert Jones splint consists of rolls of cotton wool wrapped around the broken leg. The dressing is then compressed by applying several bandages very tightly. A plastic drain-pipe, cut in half, can be added to give extra support.

Once the extent of the damage has been evaluated, the method of treatment can be decided.

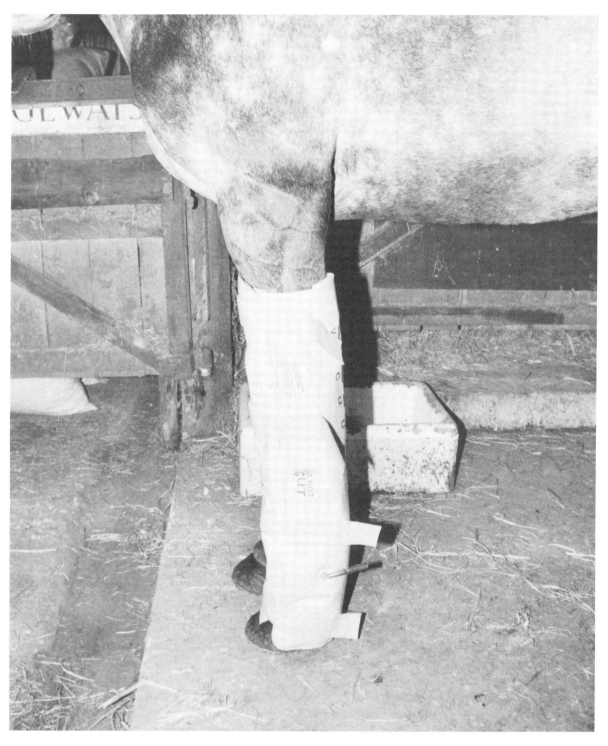

Fig 108   The vacuum splint – a new way of immobilising a limb,
borrowed from human first aid.

Treatment

The methods used to treat equine fractures can be divided into three main groups:

1.   The conservative way, where the horse is box rested, possibly with the fracture supported by an external splint. This method is of limited use, as it is difficult to obtain adequate immobilisation of the fracture site.
2.   Internal fixation is a better method. The fracture site is opened up and the fracture is aligned correctly and then fixed with screws or a plate and screws. In fractures that involve the joint, this is the only way that allows the accurate alignment which is so necessary if later joint disease is to be avoided.
3.   Small chip fractures, which often occur in the bones of the knee for example, are best treated by surgical removal.

Factors Influencing Bone Healing

Compound fractures, where the bone protrudes through the skin, and fractures that involve a joint surface, have a worse prognosis than closed fractures. Simple fractures, involving only one or two fragments, can be immobilised more effectively than a multiple (comminuted) fracture. The many fragments of this type of fracture are difficult to align and bone grafts may be needed to fill the spaces.

Young bone heals more quickly than old, but unfortunately the unaffected limbs are less able to bear the extra weight. Deformity of the overstressed bone, and overstretching of the tendons in the undamaged limbs, is a common sequel to broken bones in the foal.

The temperament of the patient is of paramount importance. The calm, placid individual is much more likely to ignore the physical awkwardness of his condition and lie down, thus relieving the strain on the normal limbs.

TENDON INJURIES

Injuries to tendons fall into two groups:

1.   Those where the tendon is partially or completely severed by external means. The serious wounds that result when a horse wraps wire around his lower leg, or when the leg is trapped between sheets of galvanised iron, are good examples. Another common cause is the overreach, where the hind foot strikes into the flexor tendons at the back of the foreleg cannon.
2.   The more common cause of tendon damage occurs when the mechanical strain exerted during violent exercise is greater than the ability of the tendon to withstand it. The damage that results can vary from rupture of just a few collagen fibres, with a minimal amount of swelling, heat and pain, to rupture of a large number of fibres. In the latter case, there is extensive haemorrhage into the tendon, the tendon sheath is damaged and the whole tendon becomes swollen and intensely painful, with a varying degree of loss of function.

Treatment

The most effective method of treating tendon injuries is complete rest during the acute phase, followed by graduated exercise during the convalescent phase. Less serious cases respond to box rest, frequent application of a cold compress (a picnic ice pack works well) and, most important, a determination not to return the horse to full work until repair is complete.

To obtain the complete rest that severe cases need, it may be necessary to apply a plaster cast. The fitting of a high heel shoe, by elevating the heel, will relax the flexor tendon and so rest it. The use of corticosteroids during this phase is helpful. They help to reduce the swelling that forces the tendon fibres apart, and also reduce the number of adhesions developing between tendon and nearby structures. Once healing starts and the swelling and pain diminish, their use must be discontinued, as prolonged treatment delays healing.

As the acute inflammatory phase dies away, to be replaced by the slower healing process, a gradual return to light exercise is permissible. The gentle forces acting on the healing tendon encourage the developing collagen fibres to lie in a longitudinal pattern, and the movement of the tendon within its sheath helps to prevent the formation of fibrous adhesions which inhibit the return to normal function. The convalescent stage is therefore a balance between exercise and pain. Any evidence of pain, and exercise must stop until the horse is sound again. As with slight tendon strain, the most important fact, when dealing with severe strain, is to realise how long the repair will take – 12 months at least.

YOUR FIRST-AID KIT

In our experience, first-aid boxes are a disaster: they always seem to be elsewhere when they are needed, and if by some miracle the box can be found, the one necessary item is always missing. However, they are an essential piece of stable equipment and can be useful too, if two rules are made and kept:

1. Always keep the box in one place, where everyone will be able to find it. Always put it back after use.
2. Replace each item as it is used and check the contents regularly to make sure that all are there.

Contents

Ideally your first-aid box should contain the following items:

1. Three or four 7.5 or 10cm bandages, conforming ones are the best. Crinx or Vet-K-Rap are two types that mould themselves to the contours of the limb very easily.
2. Two or three dressings; Melolin, or Fucidin Tulle are especially useful as both have non-stick properties. Fucidin tulle is impregnated with an antibiotic gel, and Melolin has a special porous non-stick layer which is applied to the wound.
3. One poultice-type dressing. Animalintex is a dry dressing which is soaked in hot water before use. This type of dressing is invaluable for cleaning up a dirty broken knee.
4. Scissors and a thermometer.
5. Antibiotic or antiseptic wound dressing powder. If your horse does not mind the hiss of an aerosol, this type is useful for treating minor wounds.

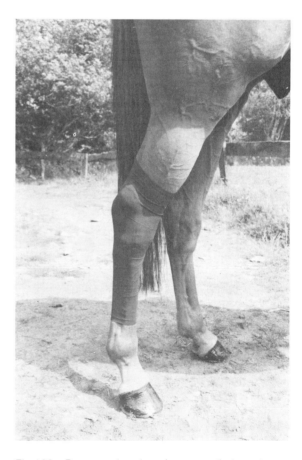

Fig 109 Pressage bandage in use on that most difficult of joints to bandage, the hock.

6. Some adhesive bandages to keep the dressing in place. Elastoplast or a self-adhesive bandage such as Vet-Rap work well on the straight part of the limbs, but if the joints are to be dressed then one of the special joint dressings such as Pressage is best. Although expensive, they are the only type of bandage that will keep a dressing in place.

7. A small bottle of cleansing liquid. Hibitane or Pevidine are both good cleansing agents, as well as being antiseptic.

8. A roll of cotton wool or gamgee. Gamgee is probably better, as its fluffy padding is covered with gauze, thus preventing the fluff from sticking to the wound.

Proprietary first-aid boxes can be bought, but more flexibility in the choice of contents can be obtained if you ask your vet to make up a box for you.

PROFESSIONAL TREATMENT

Professional advice must be sought in the following circumstances:

1. When the wound is more than an inch long and extends through the whole thickness of the skin, especially when the edges gape wide; this type of wound should always be stitched.

2. When the wound is haemorrhaging severely and cannot be controlled by a pressure bandage. This applies especially to arterial bleeding, where the blood, bright red in colour, spurts from the wound in rhythm with the heart beat.

3. When the wound is a deep, penetrating one and where the horse has not had a recent tetanus vaccination.

4. When you suspect that a bone may be broken or a tendon badly strained.

5. When a wound that was healing well suddenly develops a smelly discharge and becomes hot, swollen and painful. These signs indicate a developing infection which should

be treated without delay.

Injections

Unfortunately the cost of treating wounds and injuries is high. This is not so much due to the expense of the initial treatment, such as suturing a cut, but to the following visits that are needed, to dress the wound and administer the course of antibiotics.

One way to reduce the expense is to do these jobs yourself, but although most people feel confident in their ability to redress wounds, less are so happy about their expertise in carrying out injections. There is no need to worry. Like most procedures, there is a right and a wrong way to do it, and once the right way is mastered, injections can be given with ease and painlessly.

The first job is to fill the syringe with the drug to be injected. The easiest way to do this, perhaps for a 20cc injection, is first to inject 20cc of air into the bottle holding the drug, then, with the bottle held upside-down, withdraw the same amount of drug. Remember that it is important to use new needles each time, and to clean the plastic seal of the bottle with spirit or an antiseptic swab.

The next stage is to swab the injection site with the antiseptic and then to give the injection. Anyone who has had an injection will realise that the slow, steady approach is not always the painless one and that the more forceful approach is better. So, holding the needle between thumb and forefinger, thump the injection site three or four times with the heel of your hand, then, reversing the hand, drive the needle through the skin into the muscle. If your initial thumps were vigorous enough, the horse will not react and you can now connect the syringe and give the injection by slowly depressing the plunger, having first checked that no blood backflows into the needle. If blood appears, withdraw the needle and try again. It is unlikely that blood *will* appear, but if it does it is essential that a new injection site is found.

The most common injection you will be asked to give is an intramuscular one. This type of injection has to be given deep into a muscle mass so that the drug can be absorbed with ease and the inevitable bruising that occurs can be healed quickly. The muscle masses which should be used are those of the chest and hind quarters and *not* the muscles of the neck. The muscles in the neck are relatively thin and cover many delicate and essential structures. If, by some chance, infection is introduced through a dirty needle, the resulting abscess can cause a lot of harm and, equally importantly, the needle itself may damage these structures.

14 Current and Future Techniques

For too long the diagnosis of diseases has consisted of a clinical examination, albeit a careful and detailed one, followed by a diagnosis based on sometimes limited clinical evidence together with previous experience. Inevitably a large amount of guesswork has often been involved. In recent years, a sudden increase in research into disease conditions and their treatment has helped to provide hard evidence which can back up the diagnosis scientifically. The art and science of veterinary medicine has moved a little away from the art and towards the science. It must be stressed, however, that nothing will replace the initial, and vital, thorough clinical examination.

AIDS TO DIAGNOSIS

X-ray

X-rays have now been used for many years to demonstrate changes in bone structures of the skeleton and, to a lesser extent, soft tissue structures. A liquid which absorbs X-rays can be injected into a specific site, so that solid obstructions in that site can be delineated and identified as abnormal. For example, the technique can be used to demonstrate a constriction in the spinal canal which may affect the gait. The equipment required for such techniques is, however, sophisticated and expensive.

Scintigraphy

When we have found an abnormality, we need to identify whether it is causing the condition which we are investigating. Is a splint, for example, causing an apparent lameness in one leg? If it is, it is likely that there will be increased activity in that bone. By using a marker which is taken up by active bone and which is attached to a radioactive isotope, 'hot spots' can be located where the bone is active, using a hand held detector or even a highly complex gamma camera. Scintigraphy, as the technique is known, is still in its infancy but is potentially extremely valuable considering that more than 30 per cent of lamenesses in two and three year olds still go undiagnosed.

Endoscope

Abnormalities within spaces in the body can be visually examined using a fibreoptic endoscope which, with its powerful light source and fibreoptic system, allows examination of cavities deep within the body. Although the technique has most commonly been used to examine the respiratory tract, there is no reason why it cannot also be used to examine the urogenital or alimentary tracts.

Thermography

Soft tissues of the body can be difficult to examine but working on the principle that one of the main features of inflammation is an increase in blood supply to an area, with a consequent increase in heat, hitherto unseen inflammation can be located by measuring abnormal local increases in temperature, a process known as thermography.

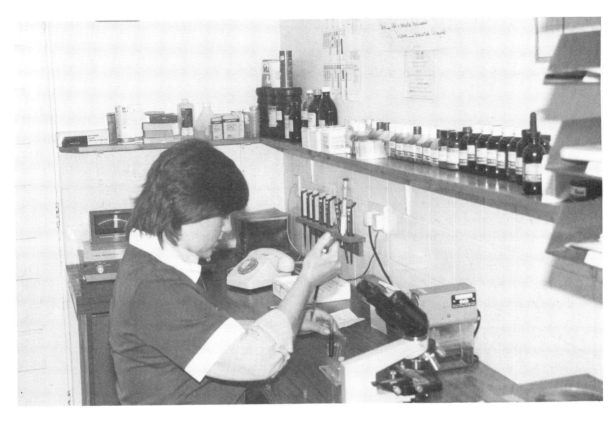

Fig 110   Laboratory back-up is an important aid to modern veterinary practice.

Ultrasound

Ultrasound is also becoming an important tool for examining the soft tissues. Currently it is directed mainly towards the diagnosis of pregnancy. High-frequency sound waves are bounced back off the tissues which differentially reflect or propagate the waves. The waves are received by a transducer and displayed on a screen. Liquid does not reflect waves and shows as a black area while dense tissues reflect as a white area. An early embryo can be demonstrated in pregnancy in the centre of a fluid-filled sac. Such pictures can be detected as early as three weeks or less into pregnancy, much earlier than by any other means. This is particularly important in Thoroughbreds where the incidence of twin preg-

nancies is high, since, if abortion is required to terminate such a pregnancy, it must be done before the six weeks at which pregnancy can normally be determined manually.

Pregnancy diagnosis is not, however, the only use for ultrasonic scanning. Various other conditions of the ovaries can also be identified, such as ovarian tumours. Diagnostic ultrasound is also used to determine abnormal size, shape, position or tissue texture of muscles, tendons, ligaments, vessels or joint capsules in the limbs, enabling a number of conditions, particularly partial rupture of tendons, to be identified.

Even some damage to the heart which is not otherwise obvious but which is significant and limits performance can be diagnosed using ultrasound.

Faradism

Damage to muscles can be identified in some cases using faradism, in which an electrical current is applied to the muscle to cause controlled rhythmical contractions. Injured muscle is more sensitive than normal. Using a rhythmical surge from a low voltage battery, graded treatment can also be used to restore normal function to damaged muscle, with a high recovery rate. If the muscle is stimulated at intervals it becomes less sensitive and lameness reduces or disappears due to the dispersal of fluid resulting from injury or, in old cases, the freeing of adhesions between muscle fibres.

LABORATORY AIDS

The laboratory is becoming an increasingly sophisticated tool to back up the clinical examination. Abnormalities in the blood cell often appear to be subtle changes in an apparently normal horse, but can be vitally important in affecting its maximum performance.

Enzymes and hormones which are responsible for speeding up chemical processes within cells are increased in the blood either when there is an increase in demand or when the cells are damaged, allowing their release. By identifying from which organs specific enzymes originate, damage to those organs can be assessed. The degree of damage can also be accurately assessed from the *level* of the enzymes.

Such examinations are not confined to blood, but can be applied to fluids taken from the bladder, the abdomen, the spinal cord and various other sites. In particular, parasites found in samples taken from the skin or faeces or washings from the lungs can give an instant diagnosis.

By growing samples on specially prepared nutrient plates under carefully controlled environmental conditions, bacteria and fungi can be identified as potential causes of disease. It is possible to identify the body's response in the blood to the presence of specific viruses, but the electron microscope allows an individual virus, tiny as it may be, to be visualised.

Samples of tissues can be removed and examined under the microscope. Obviously this is easier in a post mortem examination, but samples of various organs including skin, tumours, muscle and liver can be taken from the live horse, as biopsies, in the same way.

Finally, advancements in anaesthetic and surgical techniques have made it much safer and more feasible to reach a diagnosis by surgical exploration. Frequently, in cases of colic, for example, a diagnosis of acute abdominal catastrophe can be reached and no further progress can be made. By surgical exploration a definitive diagnosis can often be made very rapidly, and the appropriate corrective action taken where possible, or humane destruction can be performed at the earliest possible opportunity when attempts at treatment will clearly prove useless.

ADVANCES IN TREATMENT

Hand in hand with advances in diagnostic techniques has come progress in treatment. Surgical techniques become ever more sophisticated and new drugs make a continuous stream of entries into the veterinary surgeon's armoury. A trend which encourages the investigation of the underlying causes of a particular condition, and treats it from first principles, can only be beneficial.

A wealth of new ideas, largely unproven and mainly claiming to be a panacea for all orthopaedic problems, have flooded the market, engulfing those forms of treatment that are proven to be of help. Inevitably, lasers have been introduced both for cutting and destroying tissues, and soft lasers for stimulating rapid healing of wounds. Undoubtedly their use will increase.

Perhaps more encouraging is a trend to-

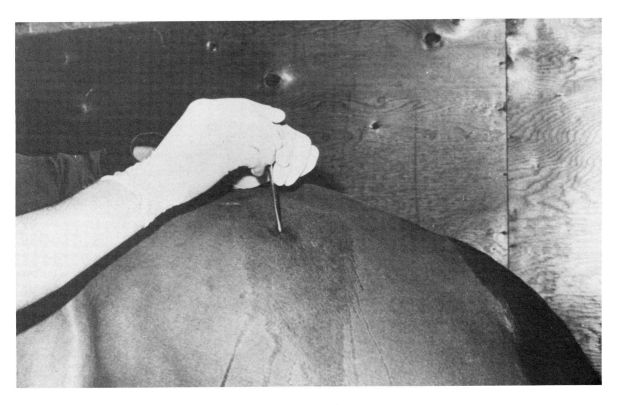

Fig 111   Taking a biopsy of muscle to assess structure and damage.

wards altering the environmental factors which predispose the horse to disease. This is most clearly evident in the respiratory diseases, where a healthy, dust-free environment is becoming increasingly recognised to be of paramount importance. In the field of orthopaedics there is increasing awareness that many lameness problems can be eliminated by having the foot correctly balanced and shod, and that many problems which do arise can best be treated following a study of the mechanics of the limb.

The horse is a finely tuned performance animal. Only by minimising disease can his maximum performance be obtained. This aim is best achieved by understanding how he functions; we can then take steps to prevent disease by vaccinating against it, or by altering the horse's surroundings to suit him so that he can function in the optimal way. The task is an infinite one, but to progress along the road towards this goal is immensely exciting.

Useful Addresses

EQUINE HEALTH ORGANIZATIONS

American Association of Equine
  Practitioners
22363 Hillcrest Circle
Golden, CO 80401

American Farriers Association
P.O. Box 695
Albuquerque, NM 87103

Animal Health Foundation
105 Carmel Woods
Ellisville, MO 63011

Morris Animal Foundation
45 Inverness Drive East
Englewood, CO 80112

Toxicology Hotline
National Animal Poison
  Control Centre
University of Illinois
2001 S. Lincoln Avenue
Urbana, IL 61801

U.S. Animal Health Association
P.O. Box 28176
Richmond, VA 23228

University of Kentucky Equine
  Research Foundation
AG-Science Building, North
Room S327 A
Lexington, KY 40506–0091

UNIVERSITIES WITH
EQUINE VETERINARY SCHOOLS

Auburn University, Auburn,
  AL 36849
University of California –
  Davis, Davis, CA 95616
Colorado St. University, Ft.
  Collins, CO 80523
Cornell University, Ithaca,
  NY 14853
University of Florida, Gaines-
  ville, FL 36201
University of Georgia, Athens,
  GA 30602
University of Illinois, Urbana,
  IL 61801
Iowa St. University, Ames,
  IA 50011
Kansas St. University,
  Manhattan, KS 66502
Louisiana St. University, Baton
  Rouge, LA 70803

Michigan St. University, East
  Lansing, MI 48824
University of Minnesota, St.
  Paul, MN 55108
Mississippi St. University, MS
  State, MS 39762
University of Missouri,
  Columbia, MO 65211
No. Carolina St. University,
  Raleigh, NC 27606
Ohio State University,
  Columbus, OH 43210
Oklahoma State University,
  Stillwater, OK 74078
Oregon State University,
  Corvallis, OR 97331
University of Pennsylvania,
  Kennett Square, PA 19104
Purdue University, West
  Lafayette, IN 47907

University of Tennessee,
  Knoxville, TN 37901
Texas A & M University,
  College Station, TX 77843
Tufts University, North
  Grafton, MA 02111
Tuskegee Institute, Tuskegee,
  AL 36088
Virginia–Maryland Regional
  College of Veterinary
  Medicine, Blacksburg,
  VA 24061
Washington State University,
  Pullman, WA 99164
University of Wisconsin,
  Madison, WI 53706

Index

INDEX